Redefining Healthcare Philanthropy

Redefining Healthcare Philanthropy

Editor Betsy Chapin Taylor

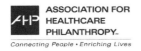

ASSOCIATION FOR
HEALTHCARE
PHILANTHROPY

Connecting People • Enriching Lives

For permission requests, please address
Association for Healthcare Philanthropy
313 Park Ave., Suite 400
Falls Church, VA 22046
ph: 703-532-6243
Email: ahp@ahp.org

Published 2014 by Association for Healthcare Philanthropy Press
Printed in the United States of America

18 17 16 15 14   1 2 3 4 5

ISBN 978-0-985321-14-7

Library of Congress Control Number: 2014940647

This book is dedicated to Bill McGinly in celebration of 31 years of leadership to the Association for Healthcare Philanthropy as its president and CEO.

His vision and service have made an indelible mark on the profession and have had a powerful ripple effect that has benefitted countless healthcare organizations.

Contents

Key Partnerships for Success

Special Leadership Topics

Foreword

William C. McGinly, Ph.D, CAE

With HEALTHCARE PROVIDERS throughout the world facing incredible challenges in delivering quality medical care and tackling issues such as access, technology, and affordability, the expectations for healthcare philanthropy have risen. In many cases, philanthropy has become central to the financial success of the healthcare enterprise.

The days of treating healthcare philanthropy as an ad hoc support system are in the past, having given way to a more structured business-like approach to raising funds. More and more development professionals are now sitting at the decision-making tables of healthcare institutions, from small rural clinics to the largest of metropolitan facilities and systems. This seat at the table calls for philanthropy professionals to be even more diligent in their work to achieve maximum impact in the communities their institutions serve and in the stewardship of their donors.

This book addresses some of the major issues surrounding healthcare philanthropy with a careful balance between both the art and the science of the profession. As philanthropy has become integral to a positive bottom line for many institutions, we have seen the profession turn to business for new approaches to increase efficiency and effectiveness. Clearly this has led to a more sophisticated and professional approach to healthcare philanthropy, but we cannot ignore the roles of relationships and stewardship. Philanthropy thrives in a culture of gratitude, and the role of the chief executive officer, physicians, nurses and other healthcare givers is more essential than ever.

In this book, chapter authors explore opportunities in the field and delve deeper into ideas that are now considered best practice. The authors are thought leaders who have pushed the boundaries to achieve excellence in this profession. As you will see from the topics they address, the strategic alignment of philanthropy with the healthcare institution, fostering a culture of philanthropy, and gaining the support of key partners are essential for a successful program.

The Association for Healthcare Philanthropy (AHP) is honored to publish this book and to acknowledge the dedication of the chapter authors, and the tireless and inspiring work of our editor, Betsy Chapin Taylor. We hope that their perspectives and experiences will serve you well in your journey as a healthcare philanthropy professional.

PREFACE

Now is our time.

Healthcare philanthropy has been elevated on the leadership agenda as a strategic revenue resource to sustain and strengthen hospitals and health systems.

At no other time in US history has the importance of healthcare philanthropy been so clear. However, with relevance comes a need for diligence.

This book brings together inspiring and challenging thinkers from across the development profession to help you explore opportunities to advance and refine your own fund development program. It is hoped this book will inspire you, enable you, and push you to achieve new levels of success and new levels of partnership.

Betsy Chapin Taylor
Ponte Vedra Beach, Florida
April 2014

Acknowledgments

THIS BOOK is the result of the inspiration and hard work of many.

This book would not have happened without the vision and support of Bill McGinly and Kathy Renzetti of the Association for Healthcare Philanthropy (AHP). AHP has been a constant driver for elevating the practice and the standards of the noble work of fund development.

This book gains its substance and resonance from amazing leaders who each agreed to share their wisdom here by authoring a chapter. These busy people from top-performing fund development organizations and consultancies gave all of us the considerable and selfless gift of their knowledge and experience.

This book gains its meaning from all the development leaders on the front line creating meaningful partnerships with visionary donors to benefit the healing work of healthcare organizations across our country.

Thanks and immense gratitude to each of you.
Betsy

Levers to Higher Performance

Develop Relationships to Accelerate Philanthropic Growth
Theresa Pesch, RN

THE US HEALTHCARE SYSTEM is undergoing tremendous change. From the ways organizations deliver care to the ways they are paid for that care, few aspects of healthcare will remain untouched. Although it might be natural to hunker down and wait for the turmoil to subside, such times can create extraordinary opportunities.

With the right approach, foundation leaders can support the path forward through accelerated philanthropic growth. Rather than focus on the challenges and obstacles, they can envision the possibilities. Strong leaders ask the question: How can our organization retool to take advantage of times of flux and transition?

Healthcare organizations that devise and execute strategic visions that support innovation, excellence, and growth as well as their mission can do more than survive these times of change; they can thrive in them. Through support from their foundation, they can take advantage of the turmoil and differentiate themselves from their peers. They can become leading healthcare systems that improve the health of the people they serve by not only delivering state-of-the-art care but also advancing it through research.

Such ambitious strategic plans from healthcare organizations, however, invariably require significant investments in capital, programming, and personnel. Few healthcare organizations have the financial wherewithal to achieve these plans out of their operating budgets or existing endowments. Instead organizations increasingly turn to their foundations to help raise money.

Of course, healthcare organizations have long relied on philanthropy, a reliance that continues to grow. But the annual fundraiser or the occasional campaign drive, while important to the organization, is not enough to create transformative change. Transformative change requires a truly robust philanthropy program that supports the strategic direction of the organization so it can accelerate growth and get ahead of the curve.

Now the question becomes: How can a healthcare organization increase fundraising at a time when philanthropy has leveled off and competition for donors has intensified? While overall year-over-year giving by individuals, foundations, and corporations rose 3.5% to $316.23 billion in 2012, giving is still well below the 2007 benchmark high of $344.48 billion, according to the latest report on philanthropy by the Giving USA Foundation and its research partner, the Indiana University Lilly Family School of Philanthropy.[1] Giving to health organizations rose 4.9% year-over-year to $28.12 billion, according to the same report.

For the answer, you must understand that successful philanthropy is no longer primarily about maximizing the size and number of transactions for any given fundraising cycle. Gone are the days when donors spread their giving among multiple organizations. Instead, they are pruning and selecting one, two, or three philanthropic organizations, and they are going deep. Fundraising campaigns are important, but the long-term success of a healthcare organization's philanthropic program depends on developing deep, meaningful, long-term relationships with donors.

People and corporations who give to an organization increasingly

---

1   Lilly Family School of Philanthropy at Indiana University, Giving USA 2013: The Annual Report on Philanthropy for the Year 2012., June 18, 2013

view themselves as investors—they want to invest their money in an organization that achieves great things or does great public good. Like all investors, they want to see positive results. This is particularly true of corporations and high-net-worth donors, who are perhaps the fastest-growing and most significant sources of philanthropy.

In other words, healthcare organizations must focus on building deep, ongoing relationships, not completing transitory transactions. When it comes to philanthropic relationships, quality, not quantity, counts most, an approach that holds significant potential.

Strategy in Action

Seven years ago, at a time when the national economy faced one of its worst recessions in decades and giving was nose-diving, Children's Hospitals and Clinics of Minnesota embarked upon a $300 million renovation and expansion project, which was supported through a $150 million fundraising campaign. Prior to this time, Children's raised approximately $4–5 million annually. Rather than take a customary approach to fundraising, the organization needed a fundamental shift to support this bold initiative. Teams and infrastructure were put in place to support the growth goals, with a new focus on establishing quality relationships to make a deeper impact. To stay ahead of the curve and leverage the latest for maximum lift, the organization worked with an organization with expertise in future healthcare trends. The result: Children's surpassed its campaign goal by 12% in just six years. Currently, the organization is raising more than fivefold annually over prior years, and it expects increases of tenfold by 2020 (less than a 15-year span).

This chapter explores specific opportunities to build a truly robust philanthropy program by more effectively engaging donors, being accountable to them, and deepening the relationships.

Building Quality Relationships

In today's uncertain economy and healthcare landscape, competition for significant donations is intense—and not just because of the need and desire of healthcare and other nonprofit organizations to raise money. Significant donors, such as corporations and high-net-worth individuals, increasingly view major gifts as part of a long-term partnership and expect thoughtful and business-like plans from potential recipients.

But first you have to identify, cultivate, and solicit donors and develop those relationships, which is no small task. Once a major gift is received, there is natural space to steward and thank the donor—it's imperative to thank more than you ask. This period should also be a time for foundation leaders to pay attention to the pipeline for long-term growth. More often than not, new donors come to the organization at the suggestion of people who are already active in the organization, such as current donors, volunteers, board members, staff members, or friends and relatives of patients.

Once donors are recruited, it's essential to create real, authentic experiences that allow them to be engaged with the mission of your healthcare organization and allow them to see firsthand the potential impact of their generosity. In many cases, donors develop into some of the best advocates for your organization and may even become members of the development committee or board. Especially if they join the development committee or board, donors must understand their own responsibilities and be given clear roles for how they can help the organization.

Today's donors think like investors and desire a relationship that goes beyond writing a check. They expect updates on the impact of their investment. "Donor-investors" also prefer to give to a specific program or goal of an organization in order to track the impact of their gift. Prior to asking for their gift, organizations should engage operations and clinicians and pre-determine how to report back to the donors and be accountable. Organizations should then work with clinician leaders to develop cases for support from hospital business plans. In this way, donors can envision where their dollars are going and see what those dollars accomplished as milestones are met.

Finally, it is critical to deepen the relationship with donor-investors, especially those who have the resources, talent, and commitment to be considered *strategic* donor-investors. Some strategic donor-investors start out in relatively small roles or by making relatively modest gifts. As relationships deepen, they begin to see a much larger role for themselves in the organization. In an increasing number of cases, these core donor-investor commitments become inter-generational.

Identify, Cultivate, and Solicit

A critical first step to any philanthropy program is to identify or recruit potential donors, and there are few recruiting tools more effective than a strong board of directors. Board members can be a healthcare organization's strongest and most influential advocates. Especially when it comes to identifying and developing relationships with strong prospective donor-investors, the most effective path is through a healthcare organization's board members. At Children's Hospitals and Clinics of Minnesota, the organization has a 70% success rate with an initial major gift from a peer referral by a board member, compared with 30% of those who come from the field.

As a result, how an organization builds and who it recruits to its healthcare or foundation boards is critical to its overall success and particularly critical to the success of its philanthropy program.

Traditionally, strong board members are considered to be those with a combination of great visibility in the community, corporate leadership, and substantial net worth. Research shows attention to wealth in board recruitment correlates with board generosity, and board generosity correlates with overall fundraising.[2] When the board gives 20% or more of what the organization raises, the organization tends to raise significantly more money than those organizations where board giving is a lower percentage.[3]

But while these criteria are important in a board member, they are not sufficient. Board candidates must have a deep commitment to supporting the mission of the hospital and have the desire to bring strategic relationships and be role models, ambassadors, and door-openers for the organization. Additionally, board members should also be ethical, generous, compatible, and willing to question the status quo. They should view their board position not as an honorary title but as a calling. They should be strong leaders and doers. Finally, the ability to recruit donors is one of a board member's most critical roles.

Just as there are new requirements for what makes a strong board member, there needs to be a new process for how that board is built. Organizations should consider a multi-year recruitment agenda that continuously looks for strong board members and volunteers. Before they are invited to join the board, there should be a period where foundation leaders get to know the potential recruits through philanthropic and volunteer opportunities to ensure they are engaged and the right fit for the board. It is better to have vacancies than disengaged board members. Term limits are set for board members, although there are opportunities for ongoing involvement.

While board members are critical to recruiting, the following are other significant recruiting tools:

Networking

It all starts with that most fundamental of business and career tools: networking. Prospective donors may already have a connection with your organization, such as a staff member, patient, or volunteer. Or they may know the organization through its work in the community.

---

2   BWF 2011 Healthcare Philanthropic Survey.

3   BWF 2011 Healthcare Philanthropic Survey.

They should be hardwired to talk about your organization from a high level and willing to invite others to be more deeply involved.

Touring the Facility

Healthcare organizations have powerful stories to tell about their mission and what they do. That's why prospective donors should tour the hospital and meet patients, physicians, and hospital leadership. In fact, nursing and medical staff are often cited as important influencers in donors' giving decisions, as are health organization executives.

Aligning Interests

Prospective donors are particularly motivated to give if they see their interests aligned with those of the healthcare organization. For instance, one donor family had a baby girl born with a diaphragmatic hernia and a slim chance of survival. The little girl spent 14 days on life support in cramped conditions with a half dozen other critically ill babies. In the end, the hospital saved her life. The mixed experience—the joy of a successful outcome combined with the discomfort of the crowded hospital room—motivated the baby's parents to become part of a significant fundraising effort to build 285 private patient rooms. The family knew firsthand how other families would benefit from private rooms. This family has also become active in other fundraising initiatives for the hospital and has a formalized and ongoing commitment to the hospital that includes helping both of their daughters understand the value of giving back.

Power of Social Media

Foundations must be present in the places, interactions, devices, and relationships that make up donors' lives, whether it be online, on the phone, or on a major social channel. Content should be developed specific to each communication vehicle. Consider hardwiring the social media team with other healthcare news to be part of the ongoing conversation.

Engagement

Donors who are emotionally and intellectually engaged in a healthcare organization are far more likely to contribute their talents, energy, and resources to that organization than those for whom the connection has faded. People desire to be, and draw satisfaction from being, a part of something meaningful.

A powerful way to engage donors—and keep them engaged—is to create meaningful experiences, such as inviting them into the health-care facility for a unique experience, where they might see a surgery, participate in a program with patients, or go on rounds. It is important that they see and experience firsthand the care that is provided. Just as touring the healthcare organization is a powerful tool in recruiting new donors and volunteers, providing renewed firsthand experiences is important in keeping donors engaged.

Besides tours, experiences may consist of:

- Home fundraising events, where a top physician may talk about new developments in a particular area of medical science;
- Peer engagement, in which donors get together to discuss a fundraising issue or work on a related task; or
- Interactions with patients and their families, which can often be the most powerful experience of all.

Another powerful piece of donor engagement is through creative, personalized stewardship and showing gratitude to donors for their gifts. For example, it can be incredibly moving to have a patient or family member write a personalized thank-you note to a donor.

When establishing major gift partnerships in particular, there is both a science and an art to successful donor engagement.

The science of engagement relates to the need for an organizational major gift and donor experience framework. Such a structure ensures board directives are aligned with strategic planning, project dash-boards, established goal measurements, and more. The organizational and major gift components then cascade into donor engagement, which provides foundation staff with the tools they need to create highly customized plans for major gift partnerships that include extraordinary experiences, donor stewardship, gift celebration, and much more.

The science framework supports the art of fundraising, which begins with getting to know the donor, including his or her background, attitudes, experiences, and motivations related to community giving and philanthropy. It also involves being open and available to form authentic, strategic, and lifelong partnerships. In many cases, it requires tapping into your own intuition and following the energy of a donor's generosity, or sensing when a donor wants to create more than a transactional gift, and leveraging those opportunities so that together you can dream about the possibilities ahead.

Using a science-and-art approach results in extraordinary relationships with donors that create one of the most meaningful experiences in their lives.

Accountability

Donors have become much more discerning about and demanding of the organizations they give to. They increasingly view philanthropy less as a *gift* and more as an *investment*. Ultimately, they want to be sure their dollars create real value and impact by giving to organizations that operate effectively and efficiently.

That's why it increasingly makes sense for healthcare organizations to think of philanthropists, especially those who make major gifts, not as donors but as allies. Likewise, healthcare organizations should view philanthropy not as a way to shore up their operating budgets but as risk capital to fund innovation and new programs. Savvy healthcare organizations ask donors to invest in a particular project or program as it aligns with the donors' interests and then report back to the donors, enabling them to track the progress—or "return on capital"—of their investment.

One effective tool is to create an individualized philanthropic history and to provide an annual personalized giving report that shows year-over-year where the individual or family has given within your organization and the impact.

This process of tying donations to specific activities, being transparent about the progress of those activities, and measuring and sharing the results of the donation not only satisfies the desire of the donor-investor to track his or her investment, but it also deepens their engagement in and commitment to the organization. That is, donors who feel their gifts are being used well and are appreciated are also likely to remain connected with the organization—and will keep contributing resources and time. Increasingly, research shows high-net-worth individuals give most to organizations where they both volunteer and believe their gift will have the largest impact.[4]

"Philanthropy is moving towards committed donors with fewer places to give," said a hospital board member. "They want fewer things to be active in instead of being involved in 10 organizations. They want to make a difference, and they want to see a difference." As a result, nonprofit organizations should develop highly customized plans to show the donors how their gift is being used and to celebrate that gift. That includes providing regular reports to the family, showing how their donation is being used.

Deepen the Relationship

Although the nation's financial picture has brightened considerably since the 2008 recession, most donors aren't revisiting the nonprofits they pruned during the recession. Instead, they are choosing to narrow and deepen their engagement with the organizations they have supported through the recession.

Healthcare organizations need to recognize this trend and take

---

4   "The 2012 Bank of America Study of High Net Worth Philanthropy, Issues driving charitable activities among wealthy households," collaboration between Bank of America and The Center on Philanthropy at Indiana University, November 2012, http://newsroom.bankofamerica.com/files/press_kit/additional/2012_BAC_Study_of_High_Net_Worth_Philanthropy_0.pdf, last accessed April 8, 2014.

advantage of it by deepening their engagement with existing donors and new donors. They also are hardwiring evaluation and metrics into the process to ensure results are measured and to show progress for major gifts. By doing so, they will be in a better position for the long term.

Given the disappointing rate at which first-time donors contribute a second time, especially considering the costs to acquire a new donor, it's essential to give thanks and show deep gratitude for first gifts to set up a more successful long-term future.

The more time a high-net-worth individual devotes to a particular nonprofit organization, the more he or she is likely to give to that organization, according to the latest research. For instance, high-net-worth individuals who volunteered less than 100 hours per year to an organization gave an average of $39,000, while those who volunteered more than 100 hours per year gave an average of $78,000.[5] In other words, the engaged high-net-worth donor gave, on average, twice as much as the one who was not as engaged.

As a result, it is more important than ever for healthcare organizations to invest more in core relationships and to grow the relationship over the donor's lifetime rather than focusing on a particular campaign cycle.

Some nonprofit organizations have come to recognize that the relationship with the donor can span not just a lifetime but generations. For example, adult parents and even grandparents bring in their kids and grandkids to contribute to a cause. To tap into this trend, some organizations create experiences that are family-friendly.

It's more than just a transfer of wealth; it's about making a difference across generations.

---

5   "The 2012 Bank of America Study of High Net Worth Philanthropy, Issues driving charitable activities among wealthy households," ," collaboration between Bank of America and The Center on Philanthropy at Indiana University, November 2012, http://newsroom.bankofamerica.com/files/press_kit/additional/2012_BAC_Study_of_High_Net_Worth_Philanthropy_0.pdf, last accessed April 8, 2014.

Consider the former St. Paul-area couple who recently gave a significant gift to complete the new neuroscience center on Children's Hospitals and Clinics of Minnesota's St. Paul campus.

Their involvement with Children's began more than 30 years ago when their sons spent time in the neonatal intensive care unit. They saw firsthand the high-quality care, commitment, and dedication of the staff, and they credited the staff with saving their sons' lives.

In the early years, the couple attended fund-raising events and regularly gave gifts to the hospital. But their relationship with Children's deepened after meeting neuroscience clinical leaders, taking tours of the hospital, and hosting fundraisers at their home. Then began the transformative years in which they opened their hearts and began to see themselves as leadership donors. Through what they themselves describe as a spiritual transformation and awakening, they recently agreed to provide a major gift.

For the future, they see themselves as true advocates for Children's, who mentor and advise, influence their peers, and make new introductions. They are introducing their family into these efforts so that the impact and relationship may become inter-generational.

Ultimately, they have come out of this philanthropic experience feeling motivated by a view of abundance and deep gratitude and awed by the ability of generosity to heal and change lives.

Conclusion

Foundation leaders must understand that while never has the future of healthcare organizations depended more on philanthropy, it is a new day in philanthropy that is full of opportunities. Foundation leaders can transform their organizations and thrive by developing donor partnerships through tailored experiences, tapping into a strategic investor mindset rooted in accountability and transparency, and providing highly customized stewardship and gratitude throughout the life-long, if not inter-generational, partnership.

Executive Summary

- Think of philanthropists as investors, not just donors; think of philanthropy as risk capital for the future.
- Be transparent, accountable stewards, and let donors see, touch and feel what they're helping to accomplish.
- Create meaningful, transparent, and real experiences that inspire donors and leave them energized.

Discussion

1. How do you work with clinical and operational teams to dream big and convey that dream to potential donors?
2. What are some authentic experiences for your donors that have worked well?
3. What are ways you have surprised and delighted your donors?
4. How do you know when you are asking too much or too often?
5. How are you creating the potential for transformational giving partnerships?

Author Bio

Theresa Pesch joined Children's Hospitals and Clinics of Minnesota in February 2007 and leads the team that launched and successfully completed the $150 million Next Generation of Care fundraising campaign, the largest capital campaign in the organization's history. By raising community support to unprecedented levels, Children's fundraising has increased more than fivefold under Ms. Pesch's leadership, which has provided the organization with resources for innovation as well as substantial facility and technological improvements. Originally trained in nursing, Ms. Pesch has 25 years of healthcare administration experience. She also serves as a faculty member of the Kaiser's Philanthropy Innovation Institute and the AHP Madison Institute. She was recognized as a *Minneapolis/St. Paul Business Journal* Women in Business honoree and is a member of Women Business Leaders of the US Health Care Industry Foundation and Women's President Organization.

Critical Success Factors in Healthcare Fund Development

William C. McGinly, Ph.D., CAE, and Kathy Renzetti, CAE

MUCH OF WHAT YOU are about to read is a compilation of the results from numerous research studies and reports the Association for Healthcare Philanthropy (AHP) has conducted over its long history. The association has analyzed, reported on, and written numerous articles and given presentations based on 29 years' worth of data from AHP's annual *Report on Giving* and various benchmarking studies identifying conclusively that the most powerful predictor of fundraising success is a foundation's total fundraising expense budget. In other words, the more your organization spends, the more your organization will raise in donated dollars.

Of course, it's not quite that simple—you have to spend your budget wisely, including hiring the right people. But altogether, investigation reveals the most influential success factors are as follows:

- Total fundraising expense budget,
- Staff size,
- Staff compensation and tenure, and
- Major gift emphasis.

For seasoned fundraising professionals, this probably comes as no surprise. Unfortunately, because of intense scrutiny faced by many fundraisers, the ability to spend money in order to raise money is no easy task. Fundraisers are questioned year after year by board members, reporters, and even executives of their own institutions about their cost to raise funds, the efficiency of their operations, and the necessity of their staffs. Fundraisers must withstand this scrutiny and see their resources cut—while at the same time being asked to raise more and more in philanthropic support.

The public's common misconception that the percentage of a charity's expenses allocated to overhead, commonly referred to as its cost to raise a dollar, is a valid way to evaluate the charity's worthiness has made it difficult for fundraising departments to grow. In many healthcare organizations, the foundation or development office is often not well understood. People don't know how it functions, the expertise its staff members must have to be successful, or the effort and expense involved in bringing in donations.

The misconceptions and gaps in understanding must change. AHP's quantitative research and statistics decisively show investing wisely in talent and compensating fundraisers fairly for their effort and experience makes all the difference in determining total net fundraising revenue and fundraising efficiency. In addition, organizations that emphasize major gifts, planned giving, government grants, and public support are the ones that show high net returns.

This chapter explains the factors that organizations should focus on as critical, shown in Figure 1, to maximize their fundraising success. It also serves as a reminder to make a priority of collecting and analyzing statistics in a standardized way to measure results both internally and externally as a profession in order to foster greater accountability and transparency.

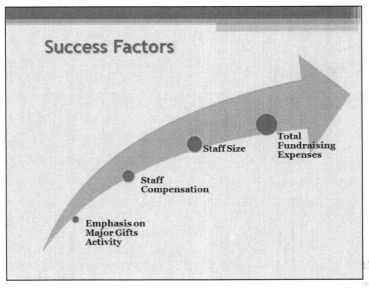

Figure 1. Based on 29 years' worth of data, AHP found these four factors are critical for highly successful fundraising.

Key Definitions and Concepts

Dealing with metrics and data can be intimidating even for the most "math-minded" among us. To fully understand the four critical success factors, it helps to be familiar with the terminology and concepts in AHP's performance-reporting standards for organizations, which are published in the *AHP Standards Manual for Reporting and Communicating Effectiveness in Health Care Philanthropy.*[6] Development professionals have been using these standards, definitions, and metrics since they were created in 2003 to provide a consistent basis for calculating and comparing results.

The *AHP Standards Manual* explains how to do the following:
- Provide a thorough accounting of all revenue resulting from direct fundraising activity,
- Calculate and attribute expenses to direct fundraising activity, and

---

6   Association for Healthcare Philanthropy. AHP Standards Manual for Reporting and Communicating Effectiveness in Health Care Philanthropy, Alexandria, VA: Association for Healthcare Philanthropy, 2012.

- Examine both projected and secured revenues to form a complete fundraising performance picture.

The *AHP Standards Manual* recommends focusing on three organizational performance metrics, which, when you look at all three together, provide the clearest picture of an organization's performance:

1. **Return on investment (ROI):** This key measure represents the financial return on each dollar spent raising funds during the reporting year. It also is the inverse of the cost to raise a dollar metric (see below). ROI is an indicator of fundraising *effectiveness,* illustrating the amount applied toward the bottom line in relation to the cost. *ROI is calculated by dividing gross funds raised by total fundraising expenses.*

2. **Cost to raise a dollar (CTRD):** A measure of fundraising *efficiency,* providing an abbreviated look at the total amount spent to raise each dollar in support of the organization's mission. *CTRD is calculated by dividing fundraising expenses by the gross funds raised during the reporting year.*

3. **Net fundraising revenue:** An important metric that reflects *bottom line fundraising revenues* for the organization or system. It is commonly described as the "what" that accompanies the "how" provided by CTRD and ROI. *Net fundraising revenue is calculated by subtracting fundraising expenses from the gross fundraising revenues that come from production.*

Production is one of two separate categories in which the *AHP Standards Manual* places fundraising revenues. The other category is Cash. When reporting fundraising returns, it is important to understand these measures and their definitions.

Cash and Production are not mutually exclusive and cannot be added together to create a single calculation of fundraising returns. Instead, they are meant to be examined as two separate metrics.

- **Cash** includes the current market value of outright gifts (made in any form) plus current-year payments from the previous year's pledges, planned gift maturities, bequests, and marketable securities. Adding these amounts together provides a picture of cash on hand, including the amount available for immediate use by the organization.
- **Production** represents all outright gifts of cash (excluding payments on pledges from previous years) and new gift commitments made in the reporting year. New gift commitments is a combination of all new pledges and letters of intent (including revocable gift commitments) and the current market value of irrevocable planned gifts. Production provides a more thorough measurement of fundraising performance than does cash and reflects the activities of the development staff.

Important formulas to calculate the measures discussed above are shown in Figure 2.

Key Metrics

$$\text{ROI:} \quad \frac{\text{Gross Funds Raised}}{\text{Fundraising Expenses}}$$

$$\text{CTRD:} \quad \frac{\text{Fundraising Expenses}}{\text{Gross Funds Raised}}$$

$$\frac{\text{Gross Funds Raised} - \text{Fundraising Expenses}}{\text{Net Fundraising Revenue}}$$

Figure 2. These formulas show how to calculate the three most important organizational performance metrics.

Avoid the "Cost to Raise a Dollar" Trap

Too many people, including professionals in the fundraising industry and volunteer leaders, fail to consider all three organizational metrics. They fall victim to the "cost to raise a dollar" trap, believing it to be the most important measure.

But a singular focus on one metric leads to poor performance. Many factors contribute to an organization's expenses, and different fundraising activities have different CTRDs. For example, organizations with a strong focus on major gifts tend to have a lower CTRD than organizations with a primary focus on the annual fund or special events.

Because such a wide range in costs and multiple variables need to be considered, it is impossible to provide one benchmark to apply across the board to all fundraising activities. Depending on the fundraising activity, an organization may appropriately spend anywhere from 12 cents to more than $1 to raise a dollar. Instead of focusing on CTRD, it is more important to consider the ROI of each activity—and to do so over a three- to five-year time frame to determine trends.

An organization's net fundraising revenue is just as important as CTRD and ROI, and as stated above, it must be considered along with those two measures for a well-rounded picture of performance. For example, you could spend $20,000 to raise $100,000, or you could spend $30,000 to raise $125,000. In the second scenario, the ROI is lower, but the net fundraising return is higher.

Many charity watchdog organizations now recognize the importance of multiple metrics and variables to measure success, and they are placing less emphasis on CTRD, as recently demonstrated in an open letter to the public from GuideStar, Charity Navigator, and the BBB Wise Giving Alliance. The letter, entitled "The Overhead Myth,"[7] denounces the "overhead ratio" as a valid indicator of nonprofit performance when viewed by itself. The letter urges donors to "pay attention to other factors of nonprofit performance: transparency, governance, leadership, and results" and points

---

7   Guidestar, Charity Navigator, and BBB Wise Giving Alliance, "It's Time to Move Beyond Overhead," news release, June 17, 2013, http://overheadmyth.com .

out that many charities should spend more on "overhead," such as training, technology, planning, evaluation, internal systems, and fundraising efforts that provide essential infrastructure and programs to enable performance.

A weak charity organizational infrastructure can lead to a multitude of problems, including inadequate staffing, financial management, and computer and support systems. Ann Goggins Gregory of The Bridgespan Group explored these challenges in an article entitled "The Nonprofit Starvation Cycle," published by the *Stanford Social Innovation Review*. The article explains that "organizations that build a robust infrastructure—which includes sturdy information technology systems, financial systems, skills training, fundraising processes, and other essential overhead—are more likely to succeed than those who do not." The article further explains how organizations "should focus on how investments in infrastructure will benefit the organization's beneficiaries, rather than reduce costs. Even within the confines of a 'cost conversion,' they should emphasize how infrastructure investments may actually reduce costs of serving beneficiaries over time."[8]

Fundraising Expenses as a Predictor of Success

AHP's findings suggest spending too little may be an indicator of poor performance. If you focus too much on keeping expenses down, your fundraising organization cannot grow.

In the *FY 2012 AHP Report on Giving*,[9] which is based on statistics reported by US and Canadian healthcare fund development organizations that are AHP members, direct human resource expenses account for the largest share of total fundraising expenses, followed by operational (overhead) and indirect human resources. Total fundraising expenses increase with the size of the institution—whether the size is

---

8   Gregory, Ann Goggins, and Howard, Don, The Nonprofit Starvation Cycle, Stanford Social Innovation Review, Fall 2009

9   Association for Healthcare Philanthropy. FY 2012 AHP Report on Giving, Falls Church, VA: Association for Healthcare Philanthropy, 2013.

determined by net patient service revenue (US), gross operating revenue (Canada), or direct fundraising full-time employees.

Over the years, benchmarking results continue to demonstrate a clear link between an organization's investment in philanthropy—that is, its fundraising expenses—and its net fundraising revenue. The data show fundraising revenue increases dramatically as expenses increase. What's more, fundraising effectiveness (ROI) and efficiency (CTRD) also improve.

Figure 3 illustrates the payoff of a strong investment in fundraising by comparing net fundraising revenue, ROI, and CTRD based on fundraising expenses. The numbers used in this comparison come from the AHP Performance Benchmarking Service.

Organizations spending between $54,000 and $503,000 over the course of the year raised $350,000 at the median level and up to $4.9 million at the top of the range. Organizations spending $2.4 million or more raised $8.7 million at the median level (nearly four times more) and almost $18 million at the top range (nearly 25 times more). Also, as you can see in Figure 3, the ROI and CTRD for those spending $1 million or more was better when organizations spent more.

Fundraising Expense Budget

The table shows the payoff of strong investment in fundraising as measured by the fundraising expense budget and median net fundraising revenue.

Total Fundraising Expenses*		Net FR Revenue	ROI	CTRD
$54k - $503k (n=13)	Median	$350k	$2.84	$0.35
	Range	$47k - $4.9M	$1.19 - $6.60	$0.15 - $0.43
$504k - $1M (n=14)	Median	$1.1M	$3.07	$0.32
	Range	$116k - $6.9M	$1.24 - $10.51	$0.09 - $0.80
$1.1M - $2.3M (n=14)	Median	$4.8M	$5.96	$0.16
	Range	$1.1M - $14.9M	$2.16 - $16.08	$0.06 - $0.46
$2.4M or more (n=14)	Median	$8.7M	$4.09	$0.24
	Range	$2.8M - $17.8M	$2.38 - $7.21	$0.13 - $0.41

Note: *Total Fundraising Expenses, Net Fundraising Revenue, ROI and CTRD, Fiscal Year 2011. Note: Outliers removed for analysis. *Fundraising expenses include costs related to direct fundraising activity, including human resources and operations expenses.*

Source: AHP Performance Benchmarking Service General Overview Report FY 2011

Figure 3. Numerical evidence of the payoff that comes from a strong investment in fundraising.

The Relationship Between Staff and Performance

The largest share of fundraising expenses is attributed to full-time employees (FTEs). Thus, it's not surprising to see the same correlation between the number of direct FTEs and fundraising revenue that we see between fundraising expenses and fundraising revenue.

Relationship between staff and performance

Direct FTE Staff Size		Net FR Revenue	ROI	CTRD
.5 - 3 direct staff (n=18)	Median	$568k	$2.98	$0.33
	Range	$47k - $2M	$1.19 - $4.58	$0.21 - $0.83
4 - 6 direct staff (n=14)	Median	$3.9M	$3.62	$0.27
	Range	$568k - $14.9M	$1.85 - $16.08	$0.06 - $0.53
7 - 9 direct staff (n=18)	Median	$5.8M	$4.21	$0.23
	Range	$1.2M - $15.5M	$2.16 – $12.76	$0.07 - $0.46
10 or more direct staff (n=15)	Median	$9.4M	$5.63	$0.17
	Range	$4.4M - $22.3M	$3.11 - $15.15	$0.06 - $0.32

Source: AHP Performance Benchmarking Service General Overview Report FY 2011

Figure 4. Larger staffs bring in more revenue—whether measured by net fundraising revenue, return on investment or cost to raise a dollar.

As Figure 4 shows, when you look at median net fundraising revenue as the leading indicator, it increases as staff size increases, hitting a high point of $22.3 million when 10 or more people are on staff. With staff sizes of seven to nine people, organizations raised up to $15.5 million. When revenue is measured by ROI and CTRD, it also improves when staffs are larger, as shown in the two right-hand columns in Figure 4.

But the relationship is not a simplistic "spend more, make more" type of dynamic. AHP's analysis shows fundraising performance is linked to the following:

- Carefully and consistently investing in the right people
  and
- Maintaining the right mix of fundraising programs
  (annual giving, major gifts, planned giving, government
  grants, etc.).

As shown in Figure 5, which uses data compiled from the AHP Performance Benchmarking Service to compare high performers (the top 25% in production) with everyone else, high performers allocate staff members to each key fundraising activity—including annual giving, major/corporate/foundation giving, planned giving, public support, and special events. At the median level (the number at the top of each row, without parentheses), the high performers have at least one FTE for each program—with the most FTEs in major/corporate/foundation giving. All others, however, have programs with no professional staff at all—as you can see by looking at both the median level and the range (shown in parentheses). Figure 5 clearly indicates that allocating adequate professional staff is associated with better performance.

High Performers - Characteristics

- ## Direct Staff Comparison

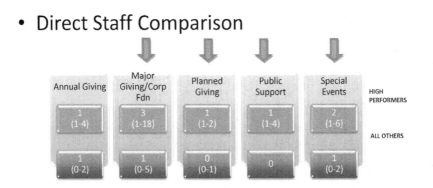

Source: AHP Performance Benchmarking Service Report II Report FY 2011

Figure 5. The top number in reach row represents the median number of full-time employees allocated to each fundraising activity. The bottom numbers (in parentheses) represent the range of full-time employees in each category, as reported to the AHP Performance Benchmarking Service in FY 2011.

Emphasizing the Fundraising Team

AHP cannot emphasize enough the importance of having a solid fundraising team. Organizations that continually rise to the top in terms of fundraising revenue, even in challenging economic years, emphasize the team and its ability to instill a culture of philanthropy. In AHP's report *Characteristics for Sustaining High Performance,*[10] the organizations studied agreed that "for the money, the right people are by far the best return on investment." When faced with budget cuts, these organizations opted to maximize all available resources in order to retain their fundraising staff. They understood the tie between the size of the development staff and fundraising revenue is real.

But the strength of the team goes beyond the donated dollars

---

10 Association for Healthcare Philanthropy. Characteristics for Sustaining High Performance, Falls Church, VA: Association for Healthcare Philanthropy, 2014

generated. AHP's report lists the top ten characteristics mentioned with high-performing teams:

4. Dedicated to the mission
5. Knowledgeable about the work and priorities of the organization
6. Smart, with good problem-solving skills
7. Team-oriented and committed to collaboration
8. Donor-centered, with focus on sustained relationships
9. Hardworking
10. Good communication and network-building skills
11. Creative and resourceful
12. Analytical
13. Focus on closing rather than serial cultivation

These teams also understand the importance of stewardship, and it is a leading priority to have a donor-centered culture in their organizations. Organizations that continually reduce staff or fail to grow staff often drop the ball when it comes to maintaining relationships with their donors. Again, from AHP's report on *Sustained High Performance*, organizations cited the importance of historically expensive programs, including:

- Stewardship,
- Donor relations,
- Campaign management, and
- Special events management and sponsorship enlistment.

Distinct Characteristics of High Performers

In its annual *Report on Giving*, AHP analyzes characteristics of institutions with the highest levels of production returns to determine the factors that affect or lead to higher performance. High performers represent 25% of all organizations reporting data for use in the *Report on Giving*. In examining the organizations who reported data for FY 2012, some distinctive characteristics emerge.[11]

---

11 Association for Healthcare Philanthropy. FY 2012 AHP Report on Giving, Falls Church, VA: Association for Healthcare Philanthropy, 2013.

US organizations

Based on the statistics from US organizations, AHP discovered the following key points:

- The median amount of production funds raised by high performers was nearly six times the median amount of production funds raised for all responding institutions: $19.1 million versus $3.2 million, respectively.
- The majority of the high performers (81.5%) had more than $2 million in total fundraising expenses in FY 2012. And median total fundraising expenses were about five times more for the high performers than for all the organizations together: $4,679,000 versus $856,097.
- Looking at overall fundraising activities (see Figure 6), high performers depended more on major gifts (31.8%) and less on annual gifts (8.4%) as major fundraising sources than did typical organizations (22.2% for major gifts and 19.5% for annual gifts).
- More than eight in ten high performers (82.4%) employed seven or more full-time direct fundraising staff.
- Fundraising employees in the organizations that employed seven or more direct fundraising FTEs were almost twice as productive in terms of median fundraising dollars per direct FTE, compared to the overall performance of all responding institutions: $1,369,653 median fundraising dollars versus $778,739, respectively.

Canadian organizations

When looking at the organizations reporting statistics from Canada, the following was detected:

- The median amount of production funds raised by high performers was nearly five times the median amount of funds raised for all responding institutions: $21.1 million versus $4.2 million, respectively.

US Production Returns by Gift Type in FY 2012
High Performers

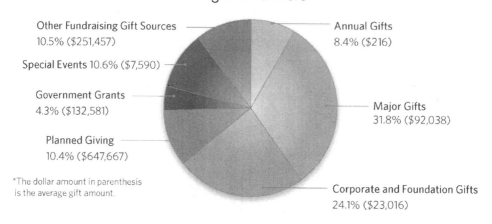

Other Fundraising Gift Sources
10.5% ($251,457)

Special Events 10.6% ($7,590)

Government Grants
4.3% ($132,581)

Planned Giving
10.4% ($647,667)

*The dollar amount in parenthesis
is the average gift amount.

Annual Gifts
8.4% ($216)

Major Gifts
31.8% ($92,038)

Corporate and Foundation Gifts
24.1% ($23,016)

All Surveyed

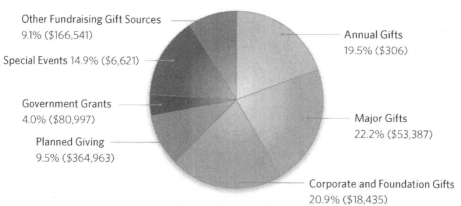

Other Fundraising Gift Sources
9.1% ($166,541)

Special Events 14.9% ($6,621)

Government Grants
4.0% ($80,997)

Planned Giving
9.5% ($364,963)

Annual Gifts
19.5% ($306)

Major Gifts
22.2% ($53,387)

Corporate and Foundation Gifts
20.9% ($18,435)

Source: AHP 2013 Report on Giving Survey

Canadian Production Returns by Fundraising Activity in FY 2012

High Performers

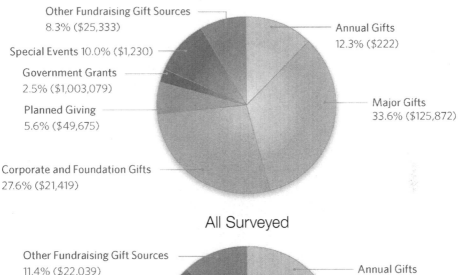

Other Fundraising Gift Sources
8.3% ($25,333)

Special Events 10.0% ($1,230)

Government Grants
2.5% ($1,003,079)

Planned Giving
5.6% ($49,675)

Corporate and Foundation Gifts
27.6% ($21,419)

Annual Gifts
12.3% ($222)

Major Gifts
33.6% ($125,872)

All Surveyed

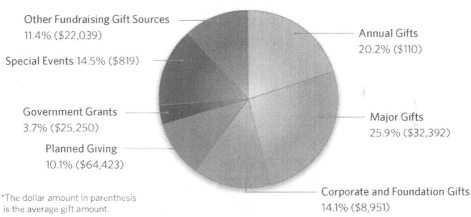

Other Fundraising Gift Sources
11.4% ($22,039)

Special Events 14.5% ($819)

Government Grants
3.7% ($25,250)

Planned Giving
10.1% ($64,423)

*The dollar amount in parenthesis
is the average gift amount.

Annual Gifts
20.2% ($110)

Major Gifts
25.9% ($32,392)

Corporate and Foundation Gifts
14.1% ($8,951)

Figure 6. AHP's statistics show that high performers have more employees and depend more on major gifts and corporate and foundation gifts than on annual gifts.

- The majority of the high performers (84.6%) had more than $2 million in total fundraising expenses in FY 2012. And median total fundraising expenses were about five times higher for the high performers than for all the organizations together: $5,233,050 versus $941,633.
- Looking at overall fundraising activities (see Figure 6), high performers depended more on corporate and foundation gifts (31.8%) and less on annual gifts (12.3%) as major fundraising sources than did typical organizations (14.1% for corporate and foundation gifts and 20.2% for annual gifts).
- More than eight in ten high performers (84.6%) employed seven or more full-time direct fundraising staff.
- Fundraising employees in the organizations that employed seven or more direct fundraising FTEs were nearly twice as productive in terms of median fundraising dollars per direct FTE, compared to the overall performance of all responding institutions: $1,780,569 versus $963,062 respectively.

Donor Pool Must Be Considered Too

An important factor that cannot be overlooked when discussing any of the performance measures defined in this chapter is the size of your donor pool. Wealth screening is specific to each organization; it is not something AHP can quantify as an overall generic metric.

Your organization needs to determine its own realistic fundraising goal based on the size and depth of your donor pool as well as your location, urban versus rural setting, type of institution, and other characteristics. Using these factors as a backdrop, you can develop your own formula—applying metrics to determine costs and to calculate your fundraising goal. Performance metrics help answer the question of whether a cost will bring a big enough return to make it worth the investment.

Lessons Learned

AHP continues to see the same four key characteristics rise to the top for high performance, which leads us to this advice:

- Make an adequate investment in fundraising, so you can develop an effective fundraising expense budget.
- Invest wisely in staff and allocate them across a mix of fundraising programs.
- Ensure that your staff is highly trained and appropriately compensated.
- Emphasize major gifts, which have been shown to bring better returns than annual gifts.
- Maintain the right mix of fundraising programs (annual giving, major gifts, planned giving, government grants, etc.).
- Systematically collect and analyze the metrics described in this chapter and present the data to your organization's executives in a way that's meaningful and easy to digest. Help them understand the role that performance metrics play in planning for success.
- Always remember the importance of stewardship and the necessity of a donor-centered organization.

Performance metrics potentially allow organizations to increase philanthropy budgets by providing empirical data to show that the investment will yield positive results. Boards and leadership teams must constantly be reminded about what solid philanthropy is and what resources you need for high performance, especially to develop a high-performing fundraising team and a culture of philanthropy that is donor-centered.

Executive Summary

- Based on 29 years' worth of data, the Association for Healthcare Philanthropy identifies conclusively that the most powerful predictor of fundraising success is a foundation's total fundraising expense budget.
- The *right fundraising staff* and the *right mix of programs* are the most influential factors for success, so these areas merit investment.
- Looking beyond the metrics, successful organizations also recognize the importance of stewardship and an organizational culture centered on philanthropy.

Discussion

1. Given the strong correlation between the number of direct fundraising FTEs and total dollars raised, balanced against hospitals' thin operating margins, when hospitals make across-the-board budget cuts including reductions in staff, does it make sense to apply the same cuts to the foundation/development staff?

2. This chapter only touches on the concept of stewardship and an organizational culture of philanthropy. Are those two concepts widely understood and implemented in your organization?

3. Does your organization measure its philanthropic impact using the three metrics discussed in this chapter: return on investment, cost to raise a dollar, and net fundraising revenue?

4. Does your organization focus too much on controlling fundraising costs? What can be done to change that approach?

5. Does your organization have the right mix of fundraising programs in addition to an emphasis on major gifts?

Author Bio

Kathy Renzetti is the Association for Healthcare Philanthropy's chief strategic officer. She has more than 25 years of marketing and communications experience and 14 years of experience with nonprofits. She oversees the development, launch, and implementation of various strategic initiatives for AHP, including government and public relations campaigns, member services, and the use of industry performance metrics.

William C. McGinly, Ph.D., CAE, is president and chief executive officer of AHP. He has more than 40 years' nonprofit management experience and has been named for 15 consecutive years in the *NonProfit Times* Power & Influence Top 50.

A Strategic Approach to Philanthropy in Healthcare

Bill Littlejohn

HEALTHCARE PHILANTHROPY has underperformed in relation to the impact of healthcare on the American economy and communities. American healthcare spending is more than 17% of Gross Domestic Product (GDP), encompassing one-sixth of the US economy, yet surveys show giving to hospitals represents less than 3% of all giving in the United States. Our glass is indeed half full; there is ample room for growth.

At the same time, US healthcare is in the most transformational era of the last five decades as major elements of the Affordable Care Act (ACA) have taken effect and the federal and state health insurance exchanges are now active. Dramatic changes in Medicare reimbursement, Medicaid funding issues, declining inpatient volumes, and the rise of high-deductible health plans are heightening threats to hospital profitability. Consolidation of healthcare institutions continues to move forward. Major rating agencies continue to project that nonprofit hospitals and health systems face an extremely challenging operating environment in the years ahead.

Globally, much is being written and presented about major trends impacting healthcare delivery—including the power of the consumer, the digital economy (including big data, wireless technology, and predictive modeling), aging demographics, and the rise of the Millennial generation. Organizations today are seeing four generations of workers.

Driven by the growth of new technologies, estimates show as much as 50% of healthcare will move from hospitals and clinics to homes and communities over the next decade. New tools such as smartphones, social media, and sensors give consumers more information and control over their healthcare decisions—and give physicians more options of where and how they treat their patients.

With these dramatic changes and uncertainty, it is more essential than ever to align philanthropy programs with their supported institutions. The philanthropy program—through its leaders, allies, and donors—is often the best vehicle to deliver the message of the value of investing in healthcare delivery and its benefit to the community.

With this backdrop and needs that far exceed traditional funding sources of earning and borrowing ahead, hospital and health system executives and boards have much greater expectations for their philanthropic programs. Too often, unfortunately, programs themselves have only been able to respond with limited success. The new model for healthcare is not fundraising but *philanthropy*—marked by the elements of best practice including strategic alignment with the institution, creating a strong and visible institutional culture of philanthropy, and focus on acquisition and cultivation of donors toward long-term and beneficial relationships. This new model requires rigor, discipline, and high expectations of performance, especially among professional staff.

It was first clearly recognized before the most recent recession and Healthcare Reform in 2008 when Moody's US Public Finance released a comprehensive brief on its rating methodology for nonprofit hospitals. Among the positive rating indicators it listed in the section on governance and management was *demonstrated fundraising ability*. Institutions involved with hospital financing, notably the bond-rating agencies, increasingly acknowledge the crucial role philanthropy can play in providing funding for hospital growth.

All of this points to the movement toward institution-based, strategic philanthropy planning. Foundations and fund development programs must conduct strategic planning processes in collaboration with institutional leadership, foundation board members, and senior staff to develop detailed short- and long-term plans, goals, and objectives. These should include multi-year revenue, expense, and funding projections as well as comprehensive cases for support that are strategically aligned throughout the healthcare enterprise. This is a dramatic departure from the annual or single-focus campaign planning that has dominated healthcare philanthropy for decades.

But how do we get there?

It begins with the understanding that a community hospital or system foundation has three primary roles:

Financial

Excellence in healthcare requires significant investment; this is achieved most effectively through a combination of earnings, borrowing, and philanthropy. Philanthropy has the power to leverage other sources of funding and creates a dramatic return on investment for donors.

Individual

The foundation facilitates the power of healthcare philanthropy by connecting grateful patients and families with caregivers, embracing the common bonds of giving and caring.

Institutional

The foundation champions and communicates the vision, plan, and case for philanthropic support for the institution. Alignment of the foundation and institution allows for effective presentation of philanthropic investment in excellence in healthcare.

Assessing Healthcare Philanthropy

The first step to develop an institutionally-aligned strategic plan for philanthropy is to conduct an environmental or comprehensive philanthropy assessment. The assessment process includes:

1. Complete a SWOT (strengths, weaknesses, opportunities, threats) analysis as it relates to the philanthropic program and its alignment with and impact on the institution.

2. Engage with key individuals (board members, executives, and physician leadership) to assess the feasibility of creating a best-practice focused, sustained philanthropic program in support of institutional capital and operational plans.

3. Conduct a thorough analysis of the institution's philanthropic program (foundations and operating entities) based on best practice models in healthcare philanthropy.

The assessment should also measure the effectiveness, efficiency, and productivity of philanthropic programs in relation to similar healthcare institutions around the country through research conducted by the Association of Healthcare Philanthropy (AHP). It is important to assess philanthropy performance from a multi-faceted perspective:

1. Measure and compare total revenue, or the actual amount of funds raised, especially over time.

2. Determine the impact of the philanthropy program as measured by its distribution of funds and participation in the institution's capital or operating budget or plan.

3. Benchmark the efficiency of the fundraising program, as measured by the ratios of fundraising costs to revenues generated.

4. Measure the effectiveness of the fundraising program in terms of the return for every dollar invested (ROI).

5. Assess the productivity of the fundraising program, as measured by the amount of funds generated per professional full-time equivalent with specific fundraising responsibilities.

A key outcome of the assessment process is the identification of Critical Success Factors, which define elements for high-performance, sustainable philanthropy within the complex environment of community hospitals and health systems.

A Comprehensive Strategic Plan for Philanthropy

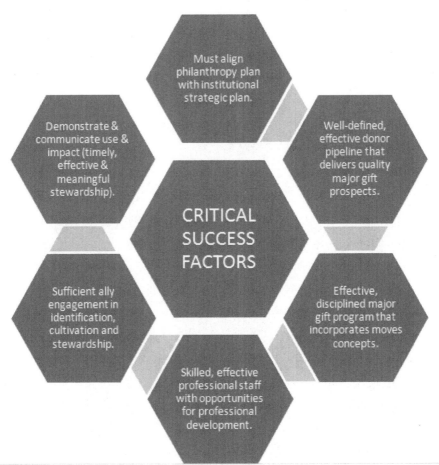

Using information gleaned from the philanthropy assessment, the second step is to prepare a comprehensive, multi-year strategic plan for philanthropy, which includes:

1. Identification of key issues and opportunities—the results of the SWOT analysis,
2. Identification of key strategies,
3. Best practice elements of the plan with short-term (two-year) and long-term (five-year) objectives,
4. Volunteer and staff organization of the philanthropic program, and
5. Detailed multi-year strategies, objectives, actions, responsible parties, timing, and measurable objectives in six key areas:
   - Leadership, governance, and strategic alignment;
   - Major and planned giving (including grants);
   - Annual giving and donor development (including special events);
   - Stewardship;
   - Physicians and philanthropy; and
   - Foundation operations.

Fundraising Components as Elements of a Strategic Philanthropy Plan

Component	Key Aspect(s)	Strategy or Metric
Leadership/ Governance/ Strategic Alignment	Institution Alignment of Philanthropy	Role of Philanthropy in the Institution; Board and Executive Roles in Philanthropy; Engagement Expectations
Major and Planned Giving (including grants)	Money	Disciplined, effective big gift process and dynamic solicitation targets; funding objectives
Annual Giving and Donor Development (including special events)	People	Acquisition, renewal, upgrade
Stewardship	Relationships, Stewarding of Money and People	Retention, Loyalty; Impact of Philanthropy
Physicians and Philanthropy	Physician Engagement in Philanthropy	Physician Engagement: as donors and champions who refer grateful patients and families
Foundation Operations	Efficiency and Effectiveness; Professional Development	Centralization, Benchmarking; Five big measures: Revenue, Impact, Cost, ROI, Staff Performance

Health System Considerations

With the continued growth and development of healthcare delivery systems, the strategic plan for philanthropy needs to respond accordingly. A colleague once remarked that Association for Healthcare Philanthropy (AHP) member institutions are like snowflakes; no two are alike. This is especially true for healthcare systems, so the philanthropy plan has to be very closely aligned with the system structure. Unfortunately, and for a myriad of reasons, the philanthropy program is often last to be incorporated or aligned in an overall system plan.

Two key elements in a health system philanthropy plan are the role of the system board and/or executive leadership in philanthropy and the centralization of philanthropy functions for efficiency and effectiveness. At the same time, major gift philanthropy must be grown and maintained across the enterprise. The degree of centralization is dependent on the primary focus of the philanthropic program in cultivating individual relationships.

To review, a strategic plan for philanthropy for a health system will need to incorporate and integrate the following four major elements:

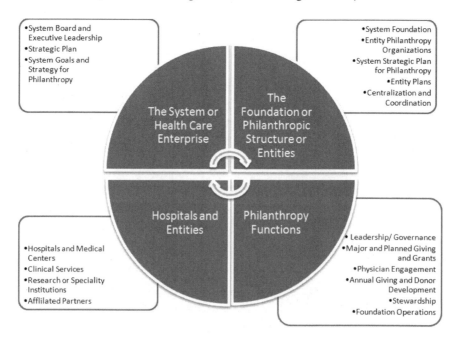

A strategic plan for philanthropy for a hospital or health system is critical as the maturity and maximum effectiveness of the philanthropic program will take several years to fully achieve:

- **The first two years** must focus on foundation structure (including the system foundation and hospital governance and relationships), strategic plan development, systems and standards of practice, recruiting and orienting staff, institutional strategic alignment, case building and grateful patient donor and prospect pipeline development at the entities. During the first two critical years of system program development, the following should be included:

Infrastructure Issues
- Determine the board and committee structure of the institutional philanthropic program.
- Establish and define the role recruitment of a senior officer for philanthropy.
- Define foundation and entity volunteer and staff leadership roles in the philanthropic program.
- Develop a strategic plan for philanthropy for the system.

Alignment Issues
- Develop multi-year, system-wide (consolidated from entity-specific) revenue, expense, and funding projections and comprehensive cases for support that are strategically aligned with the system and entities and supported by the foundation and philanthropic structure.

Performance Issues
- Develop best practice models in philanthropy functions, including both entity-focused programs (such as major gifts, special events, and stewardship) and system-focused (such as planned giving, grants, database management, asset management, and donor and prospect research).

- **Years two through five** must focus on continued donor acquisition and relationship development, stewardship of initial donors and funds, expansion of institutional ally engagement (boards, physicians, executives), major donor and prospect pipeline development, and focused major gift initiatives.
- **By year five,** the philanthropic program should be oriented around long-term, sustained, major gift development with robust acquisition, a solid donor pipeline, and a well-defined "big gift" dynamic that is enhanced by an upgraded stewardship program.

The single most important element in a major healthcare philanthropy program is the chief development officer. This chief executive leads the foundation, serves as the principal gift officer, and participates as an active and engaged member of the senior management team. This is important because senior hospital and health system managers must play a critical role in educating system and foundation board members and community donor prospects on:

- the excellence of the health system and its member institutions,
- the challenges it faces,
- how it is addressing the challenges,
- the need for philanthropic support, and
- specific projects and initiatives.

This role is particularly important in the current healthcare environment when donor publics—including board members—are confused by changes in the healthcare system and their local hospitals.

Initiative-Based Philanthropy and Comprehensive Campaigns

In alignment with the institutional strategic direction and in collaboration with system leadership, foundation board members, and senior staff, the foundation can move to strategic, initiative-based, major gift philanthropy and a comprehensive campaign. The foundation can develop detailed short- and long-term plans, goals, and objectives, including three- to five-year revenue, expense, and funding projections as well as a comprehensive case for support that is aligned with the strategic plan and the financial needs of the institution. The result of this plan will be multi-year philanthropy initiative targets or goals and the validation of the importance of philanthropy to the institution. Philanthropy will, therefore, support the continuation of patient care programs throughout the community, as well as directly fund capital acquisitions necessary for both ongoing operations as well as strategic investments in technology, programs, and innovation. The plan will demonstrate the strong link between financial and philanthropic success and the ability to fund strategic investments. The plan is contingent upon strong operations, implementation of strategic initiatives, and fundraising, all of which are necessary in an era of healthcare transformation.

Initiative-based philanthropy is a cornerstone of comprehensive campaigns and is, again, tied to institutional strategic plans and objectives. In a comprehensive campaign, initiatives can support the overall healthcare system, an individual hospital entity, or a program or function and can incorporate one or more funding objectives, such as:

- capital,
- technology and equipment,
- program development and support,
- research and education, and
- workforce support, including scholarship and endowment.

Since one of the critical success factors is the involvement of leadership allies to include physicians, executives, and board members, a comprehensive campaign presents a significant opportunity to develop enterprise engagement. The success of any healthcare philanthropy program is highly dependent upon engagement across the healthcare enterprise to include executives, physicians, staff, and board members as well as those the healthcare organization serves.

Major gift training and development has frequently been built around the concept of being "donor-centric" for good reason. Major gift success comes from strong and powerful relationships between the donor and the institution that are often facilitated by philanthropy professionals. Yet what makes healthcare philanthropy unique is that the impact and influence of allied relationships on donors are most often a result of the healthcare experience. We must be "ally-centric" in our roles as well.

Creating a successful, comprehensive campaign therefore requires the identification and engagement of initiative champions and the development of aligned funding objectives. Such a plan could include the following grid:

Initiative	Primary Location	Funding Target	Physician Champion(s)	Executive Champion(s)	Volunteer Champion	Foundation Staff Lead
Capital Initiative						
Technology Initiative						
Program Initiative						
Research Initiative						
Endowment Initiative						

The Sharp HealthCare Experience

Sharp HealthCare is a nonprofit community asset created by the people of San Diego for the people of San Diego, and it is the largest regional integrated healthcare delivery system in the county. Today Sharp HealthCare touches the lives of approximately 800,000 people each year and operates on the premise that nonprofit hospitals can better serve their communities when linked through a well-managed, integrated system of healthcare services. Sharp was a recipient of the 2007 Malcolm Baldrige National Quality Award, which is the nation's highest presidential honor for quality and organizational performance excellence. Sharp HealthCare is supported by three nonprofit philanthropic foundations.

Philanthropy is at the very heart of what Sharp has achieved to-date and aspires to accomplish for the community.

Philanthropy is a key component of Sharp HealthCare's strategic planning process. Each year, a five-year financial projection is performed. The resulting five-year plan provides the financial direction for the organization and serves as a feasibility analysis by quantifying the financial impact of Sharp's strategic initiatives.

The philanthropic component of the Sharp HealthCare's Five-Year Operating, Cash, and Capital Plan is a nationally recognized best practice; over the last decade, the Sharp Foundations have provided more than $140 million *in cash* to the five-year plan, leveraging a billion dollars in investment. Combined, the Foundations fund 10 to 15% of Sharp's capital expenditures annually; such donations support the continuation of patient care programs throughout the system, as well as directly funding capital acquisitions necessary for both ongoing operations and strategic investments.

Overall, the plan validates that Sharp's capital initiatives are feasible and that continual improvement in Sharp's financial position is expected. The plan is relied upon by Sharp's outside rating agencies, Moody's Investors Service, and Standard & Poor's in their evaluation of Sharp's financial strength and growth over each five-year horizon.

Telling Our Story

Healthcare is being transformed like never before, and philanthropy is and can be a driver of transformation. Fund development executives must embrace change and reshape philanthropy programs—not built on the concept of need, but on achieving an institutional vision and inspiring a better future.

A powerful dynamic of philanthropy is the concept of legacy. But all too often, legacy becomes "we've always done it this way" in campaigns, events, board meetings, and communications. It's time to create a new legacy for healthcare philanthropy.

An aligned strategic plan for philanthropy provides the road map for what development organizations often do best: tell stories. Stories of hospitals adapting to change and empowering their workforce. Stories that demonstrate the miracles of modern medical technology. Stories that share how healthcare organizations help families navigate an unfamiliar world. And, above all, stories of inspired giving—giving that transforms lives, institutions, and communities.

This means development leaders need to be at the forefront of writing their own stories: the case for the transformation of healthcare through philanthropy. These stories also need to be shared through a myriad of platforms, with a variety of groups and stakeholders, and across generations.

Campaigns are successful because they do two things well: They ask enough people capable of giving, and they do it in the most effective way. Strategic planning for philanthropy allows development leaders to create stories of the power of philanthropy to transform healthcare and lead the way in creating a stronger future.

Share Your Story through Your Plan

1. Begin with an institutional commitment to the power of philanthropy to transform healthcare in your community.
2. Assess your philanthropy program.
3. Define the critical success factors for high performance and sustainability.
4. Engage the enterprise in plan development.
5. Align the institution vision and plan with a plan for philanthropic investment.
6. Go back to the beginning—demonstrate the power of philanthropy to transform healthcare!

Executive Summary:

- The new model for healthcare is not fundraising, but *philanthropy*—marked by the elements of best practice including strategic alignment with the institution, creating a strong and visible institutional culture of philanthropy, and focus on acquisition and cultivation of donors toward long-term and beneficial relationships.
- Foundations and fund development programs must conduct strategic planning processes in collaboration with institutional leadership, foundation board members, and senior staff to develop detailed short- and long-term plans, goals, and objectives.

- Foundations should assess their own work to measure the effectiveness, efficiency, and productivity of philanthropic programs in relation to similar healthcare institutions around the country.
- A strategic plan for philanthropy for a hospital or health system is critical to ensure maximum effectiveness of the philanthropic program.
- It takes communication, collaboration, and commitment across the healthcare enterprise to move to strategic, initiative-based philanthropy.

Discussion

1. Is your healthcare enterprise currently strategic in its approach to alignment and coordination between the hospital or health system and the philanthropy endeavor?
2. What are the critical success factors for high performance and sustainability in your organization? How can you pursue, refine, or leverage those aspects of your work?
3. How could you foster enterprise-wide, strategic alignment between your healthcare organization and your philanthropic organization?

Author Bio

Bill Littlejohn is one of the nation's leading healthcare philanthropy professionals. With three decades of experience, Bill has led and directed philanthropic programs that have generated half a billion dollars. Bill joined Sharp HealthCare in 2002 as Senior Vice President and Chief Executive Officer of Sharp HealthCare Foundation. He oversees the entire philanthropic program for Sharp, San Diego's largest healthcare provider and recipient of the 2007 Malcolm Baldrige National Quality Award. Under his leadership, Sharp has generated nearly $200 million in philanthropy. Bill earned a degree in economics from the University of Virginia. He is 2012–2014 Chair of the Association for Healthcare Philanthropy.

Making Your Case Statement a Passion Paper

Jan Wood

BOARDSOURCE, a national consulting group that advises nonprofit organizations on a myriad of board development and governance issues, defines a *case statement* in the following way:

> *A case statement is a document that provides the rationale and justification of a fundraising effort. It can make a case for a specific program or project, or it can advocate for general operating support. It focuses on a dilemma that needs to be fixed and explains the organization's proposed resolution.*[12]

Although that is an accurate technical description of a case statement, it is missing the two most important things that make any case statement successful: passion and inspiration. Certainly a case statement needs to have strong technical and factual support to provide the justification for the need and, therefore, the request. Donors are in many ways investing in the cause at hand, and those investors want to

---

12 From the web site for Grant Space—a service of the Foundation Center. http://grantspace.org/Tools/Knowledge-Base/Funding-Research/Definitions-and-Clarification/Case-statements

know their gift will be used in thoughtful ways and that the results of those investments will be carefully measured to have the largest possible positive impact.

But most donors, especially at the major gift level, give out of passion for a mission and inspiration about a vision. Donors are motivated by more than facts, figures, and justifications. They are inspired by visionary discourse that paints a picture of a better world that will result from their support of the program or project at hand.

In reality, few fund development leaders want to see themselves as arguing a case or persuading someone to do something. That's a lawyer's job, not a fundraiser's job. The giving officer's role is to help donors identify and achieve their dreams, to help them make a mark on their world that brings them pride and personal fulfillment, and to tap into their passions that inspire them to make an impact.

No one can deny the importance of the mechanics of creating the statement itself. Those mechanics support the tone and ensure a donor feels confident about the validity of the dream or vision and its ability to truly yield results that have real impact. But a successful case statement is much more than an intellectual, cerebral communication tool. It is a "passion paper" that, like the act of giving itself, touches the heart and the imagination.

Constructing the Case Statement

The elements of a strong case statement go back to the basics: *who, what, when, where, why,* and *how.*

In a strong case statement, the *why* actually plays two roles. The statement must address: 1) why this program or initiative in question is needed and 2) why the program or initiative will make an impact.

Let's start with the first *why,* which often relates to what is happening in healthcare at the time. As much as any economic sector, healthcare is very dynamic. Economic forces, technology, and scientific discoveries all impact and change how care is delivered and financed. It is in this sea of unrest that donors need to understand the first *why* of the current state and foreseeable future of healthcare, creating a need for or the right opportunity for this initiative.

This is where the stage is set, talking about healthcare and the community needs that create the imperative for the program or initiative proposed. At this stage, it is important not to be too esoteric or generic in the *why*. Donors must be able to relate to the need in order to feel the passion discussed above. Although the need and the impact may indeed have universal implications (this is especially true when making a case for research funding), it is critical to bring the message home. The donor needs to be able to relate to the *why* and feel a personal connection on some level. The case may talk about heart disease being the number one killer in the US, but it must then bring the message down to the human level: "In the next year more women in our community will die from heart disease than from all cancers combined."

Once the stage has been set to describe the reason for the need, the case must state the *what*—what exactly is the program, initiative, service, facility, or equipment that is needed. Here, several questions need to be answered:

- Does this have a track record of success (it is improving care at other hospitals, and therefore we should have it here), or will this initiative break new ground?
- What is new about this? How will it change and improve how care is currently provided for patients and families?
- What challenges face us if we do not do this? What risk do we face if we do not secure the needed funding?
- What challenges face us if we do move ahead, and how is the team preparing to meet those challenges?

More than any other area within the case statement, the *what* section needs to use language that evokes passion and inspiration in the prospective donor. It must tie back to people and clearly illustrate the difference this initiative will make in the lives of patients and families. At their core, virtually all donors want to know they are improving lives in some way.

Always remember the *so what* test. Ask the question, "If we don't do this project, so what?" If the answer is not compelling and passion-provoking, the case will not be strong enough to yield results.

This should lead the case statement to the second, and most significant, *why*: why this is important. This is a pivotal point in the case statement that brings the conversation back to the most basic level—care for people who need it. The *why* here may head in a variety of directions that range from community need to treatment breakthroughs to workforce development. No matter what the case is supporting, this is the time the focus must come back to the benefit for people and whether that benefit is for patients and families or for caregivers.

In building a strong case, it is important to establish the credibility of those who are responsible for the initiative being a success. For example:

- Is the research being conducted by a leading physician?
- Is the facility being designed by a nationally recognized architect?
- Was the program conceived by a team of caregivers with an exemplary record of care?

It's an old fundraising adage: people give to people. Similarly, people invest in people; so it is important to communicate the credentials, expertise, and commitment of those who will bring the vision to life.

The *who* of a case statement is also related to the importance of testimonials from people who can speak from experience and from the heart about the initiative. Testimonials take the subject matter from an intellectual discourse to an emotional level. As patients, physicians, nurses, and caregivers share their personal stories, the donors begin to clearly see how this initiative, and ultimately their gift, will truly impact lives in a meaningful way. In a strong case statement, it is important to spread the testimonials throughout the document and ensure a diverse (age, patient/family/caregiver, geography, medical condition/need, race, etc.) range of perspectives are represented. Testimonials to which donors can relate or with which they can empathize prove to be the strongest and most effective.

One of the most difficult challenges of any case statement is to find the balance between inspiring the reader and managing expectations. Where is the line between passion and "over-selling"? The *when* represents an area where the reader's expectations must be managed. This is especially true when looking for funding for research or other initiatives with a long time horizon, where the donor may not see the impact of her gift for years.

In this case, the language must convey a future focus and describe a vision for someday, rather than describing an if-then proposition. The if-then proposition conveys a shorter time horizon and often is built on a sense of urgency: "*If* funding is secured for this new hospital pavilion, *then* the hospital can open a gerontology unit to care for the area's aging population." It is vital to determine whether the project in the case statement warrants a futuristic vision or a sense of urgency.

Timing has an interesting impact on another component of the case statement—the issue of *where* the initiative will take place. As recently as five years ago, the issue of *where* was relatively simple. Initiatives most often were designed to take place somewhere in the hospital. However, with the advent of Accountable Care Organizations and population health, more and more care and programs are designed to take place outside the walls of the hospital.

This is a new concept for many donors, especially those who have a long history of giving to an organization. Therefore, the *where* is not as simple as it used to be and requires greater finesse and explanation. Beware not to get sidetracked at this point in the case statement and run the risk of losing energy. A discussion of where care is provided could become complex if it is for initiatives such as community clinics or telemedicine. Here it is important to give the reader enough information to conceptualize the care delivery model, but be careful not to get mired in the details. This section should be the briefest in the case statement, if possible, so as not to slow the building momentum.

At this point, it is time to answer the question of *how* the subject program, initiative, or capital need can be achieved. This is the call to action. Although there are many effective ways to position the need for funding, one particularly effective method includes detailing examples of what gifts at different levels could make possible. By detailing how gifts from $10,000 to several million dollars can make an impact, the case statement provokes passion that the reader can attach to an outcome or impact that she finds inspirational. This is where it is important to paint a picture in such a way that the reader sees herself as part of the effort.

Engaging Key Stakeholders

Once the draft of the case statement is complete and has been blessed by organizational leadership, the statement needs to be tested and refined. If done properly, the testing phase becomes the ideal opportunity to begin securing potential donors, both from the pool of past donors and from a list of donor prospects.

The best means for this testing is through the use of focus groups: one for current, leading, loyal donors and one for donor prospects. These are not formal focus groups with one-way glass, administered by a professional focus group company. Rather, these are informal focus groups run by the development staff, where key constituents are asked for their opinions and feedback regarding the case statement. If done properly, this sets the stage for both the private and public phases of the campaign, as explained below.

Each focus group should be comprised of 10 to 15 people who fit the respective category (loyal donor or top prospect). The focus group participants should be invited by a personal telephone call or visit to explain the project and detail why they would provide valuable input to this effort. This is an excellent opportunity to begin to position the eventual request with the donor or prospective donor by detailing the vision of the campaign and getting them interested in it at an early stage.

Once you have the group finalized, send a draft of the case statement to each member one week prior to the focus group meeting and ask them to review it carefully and come prepared to share their thoughts and recommendations. Remind participants this is a confidential document that is not to be shared with anyone else.

The focus group should last no more than 90 minutes. The agenda should focus on garnering feedback on key elements of the case statement, including the theme, the tone, the case itself (what, if any, aspects of the case do the participants feel are truly compelling?), and the call to action (too strong, not strong enough, etc.). Throughout the 90 minutes, ask each member of the group to not only critique what they have read but also to offer suggestions for making the case stronger.

Listen carefully.

If the right questions are asked, donors and prospective donors will clearly communicate (directly or indirectly) if they are motivated to support this campaign, what aspect of the campaign should be proposed to them specifically, and at what level they are interested in participating. This is where focus groups lay the groundwork for some of the first donor requests in both the public and private phases of the campaign.

There should be two forms of follow-up from the focus group. The first is a letter from the Foundation President and the hospital or health system CEO, thanking the donor for participating and explaining how vital his or her role has been in shaping the direction of this effort. The second is a copy of the final case statement (before it becomes public, to reinforce the donor's feeling of being an insider) with a cover letter thanking the donor for being a "founder" of this campaign. If done well, these two steps will enhance the donor's feeling of ownership in and commitment to the effort.

Once the focus group process is complete and the second draft of the case statement is written, it is time to engage a designer to bring the document to life visually. The design of the case statement needs to effectively capture and communicate the key theme and tone of the campaign, yet it also needs to align with the organization's brand. This means involving the marketing and strategy team in the design phase to ensure adherence to the organization's brand standards. Anyone should be able to see this statement and know almost immediately to which organization it is connected.

Once the final draft is complete in mock-up format, it should be distributed to key members of the leadership for feedback and buy-in. This distribution list includes, but is not limited to:

- The organization's CEO and "Cabinet"—chief medical officer, chief operating officer, chief nursing officer, chief financial officer and chief strategy officer;
- The executive committee of the foundation board;
- Key physician leaders, especially the chiefs and/or medical directors of the service lines included in the case statement;
- Key nursing leaders, especially those leading the nursing for the service lines included in the case statement; and
- Any other leader (administrative or clinical) whose help you will need when presenting to donors once the campaign is in full swing. Like the focus group participants, these people need to feel a sense of being an insider and a sense of ownership in order to be effective partners during the active phases of the campaign.

Remember too many cooks in the kitchen can be dangerous, and editing by committee is never effective. Therefore, leaders reviewing the final draft must be clearly instructed on their role in the process, namely reviewing for factual accuracy and/or identifying any pieces of the case statement that are in potential conflict with the direction of the organization's clinical program. Be grateful if a reviewer catches a typographical error, but do not encourage "wordsmithing" of any kind other than for accuracy's sake.

Once the case statement is produced in its final form, present it to both the healthcare organization's governing board and to the foundation board, as well as the organization's top leadership. These key leaders should see this important document before it is shared outside the organization for donor meetings or any other public purpose.

Remember a case statement is a living document that will likely have a shelf life. Therefore, review the case statement annually to ensure that it is still accurate and relevant. If necessary, produce a statement supplement that keeps the document current.

Although every case statement, like every organization, is different, there are universal opportunities to add strength to the final product:

- Clearly think through the characteristics of the reader and align the message to those characteristics. If this is a case statement for a new initiative that will take the organization in a new direction, chances are that potential donors may be new to the organization and less familiar with its history. This means a portion of the case statement will need to educate these donors on the organization itself, especially its mission, vision, and values, along with its most noted accomplishments. If the case supports expansion of an existing program, service, or facility, the reader will be likely be very familiar with the organization and not need this additional education.

- Visuals make a difference, and they should focus on people rather than on charts and graphs. The most effective case statements tie the message back to how the initiative will make care better for patients. Use visuals that depict this hands-on care. Graphs spark the intellect, while photos inspire passion and emotional response.

- The case statement should not tell the entire story—that is the job of gift officers and volunteers. An effective case statement should give enough information to evoke an emotional response from the reader and inspire more thought about the initiative. If given to a donor prior to the in-person request (this is NOT recommended, but it happens) the case statement should cause the reader to formulate questions for their meeting with the development team. If given along with the proposal and letter of intent at the end of the donor-request meeting (the ideal use), the case statement should reinforce the discussion from the donor meeting and prolong the donor's excitement about the organization and the initiative itself. Never try and tell the whole story in the case statement. It is virtually impossible to do this well, and it diminishes the need for the personal visit with the donor, which is always the most appropriate and effective method for major gift fundraising. A case statement is *nothing more than a tool* in a large tool box. It supports the major giving process, but it does not qualify *as* the major giving process.

A well written case statement is a powerful tool in major gift fundraising, and a poorly prepared case statement can quickly deflate the enthusiasm of a potential donor. However, at the end of the day, fundraising is about people, passion, and relationships, and nothing replaces the power of a meaningful personal connection.

Executive Summary

A strong, thoughtful case statement is a valuable tool in any campaign effort. It sets the tone and theme for the campaign, and its development provides an ideal means for pre-campaign cultivation of key constituencies. At the end of the day, there are three key points to remember to optimize the effectiveness of any case statement:

- Giving is about passion and inspiration. Although factual support and justification is vital to any strong case statement, the case statement will not be compelling to the donor or successful for the campaign if it does not clearly and enthusiastically communicate the passion and inspiration of the initiative. What is the impact on people? How does this truly touch and improve lives? How does it transform the way we provide care?
- Use the case statement development process as an effective pre-campaign cultivation tool. Including the right loyal

donors and top donor prospects in the process allows for early buy-in to the effort, while it also enables the fundraising team to identify successful strategies for these individual donors. In short, it allows for accelerated seeding of the campaign.

- Secure internal buy-in before a case statement is finalized. Key organizational leadership will be invaluable in the presentation of the campaign to potential donors. If these leaders do not feel a sense of passion and confidence in the case, they will not be effective partners in the cultivation and solicitation process.

Discussion

1. Learn from success. What two to three successful campaigns have you admired for their success and their message? Secure a copy of their respective case statements and review them. Did the case statement inspire passion in the reader, rather than arguing the case? Did the case statement make you want to learn more about the project? What made you feel connected to the message—the visuals, certain phrases, the testimonials?

2. What is the unique selling proposition, *i.e.*, why is the request compelling and unique in your community? What need will this fill that no other organization can fill as well? Why is the organization uniquely positioned to optimally meet this need?

3. What obstacles will be faced with this campaign? Is there enough evidence to meet the intellectual requirements for a strong case statement? Is the subject matter compelling on an emotional or inspirational level? Just because a need exists, it does not mean that it will be appealing to donors. Does the request truly have what it takes to inspire passion in current and prospective donors?

4. Be sure to work with administrative and clinical leaders
    of the initiative to understand the timeline and specific-
    ity of the funding need. Is this an initiative that is clearly
    defined or is it one that may evolve over time? If the
    latter, keep the case statement somewhat open-ended
    and visionary rather than prescriptive. This will give the
    document a longer shelf life and allow the team leeway
    to grow the initiative organically without being chained
    by commitments made to the donors.

5. Finally, is this an opportunity to bring a new breed of
    donor into the organization? Think creatively and stra-
    tegically about who might support the initiative. Can
    this effort be used to attract and inspire new donors for
    the organization, rather than simply relying on the tried
    and true? If so, does it make practical and financial sense
    (depending on the budget and size of the campaign) to
    produce two versions of the case statement—one for exist-
    ing donors and one designed to attract a new group of
    donors to the organization? For example, is this a pedi-
    atric initiative where the donor base can be enlarged to
    attract much-needed younger donors who can grow the
    organization's donor base and be groomed to be major
    donors in the years ahead?

Author Bio

Jan Weinberg Wood is president of the Anne Arundel Medical Center
Foundation and chief development officer of Anne Arundel Health
System. For more than three decades, she has worked with a variety of
nonprofit organizations, leading initiatives in fundraising, marketing,
strategic planning, and public relations.

A New Major Gifts Strategy that Offers, but Doesn't Depend on, Hope

Steven A. Reed

He HADN'T PLANNED on having this conversation.

It started casually in the hallway at a conference. Now, he found himself baring his soul to—of all people—a performance improvement consultant.

As the conversation progressed, Joseph[13] heard himself becoming more and more candid. His deep-seated—but, until now, unspoken—concern about the performance of his fundraising organization was coming out.

"We've tried to put more emphasis on major gifts and have added another major fundraising event," he was saying. "We're just having trouble getting the board and our campaign volunteers energized. Nothing seems to be making a difference."

"Is it us? Is it the economy? Or has something fundamentally changed?"

Joseph's most secret fear is that maybe, just maybe, he had grown his fundraising operation to a size that exceeded his market capacity.

---

13 The story is a bit of a composite, but entirely true. The names have been changed and details disguised to protect the innocent.

The next day, Susan—head of a nine-person shop that raised an average $3 to $4 million annually—voiced a different concern. "I know we should be raising more money, and I know we're not getting our share of major gifts," she said. "How do I get to the next level when my budget gets squeezed every year?"

Susan's most secret fear is being boxed-in and never able to achieve the level of performance that she knows is possible in her market, is needed by her hospital, and is her professional ambition.

Few of us feel raising money is becoming easier. Yes, giving increased by 3.5% in real dollars in the last reported year.[14] At the same time, there's evidence we may be experiencing a "new normal" that is a much tougher environment than that of past decades. Giving overall is still down 8% in inflation-adjusted dollars from where it was in 2007.[15]

Clearly we face change. And maybe we face some fundamental shifts in donor expectations and how donors give. But despite Joseph's secret fear about his market potential, the constraints to fundraising performance are primarily internal, and *hope* too often remains the principal strategy.

In this chapter, you will explore the Four Pillars of Performance Improvement as well as the *connector, maven,* and *closer* team concept and a stage-gated major gifts process—ideas that are part of a new approach based on Lean Six Sigma thinking to improve healthcare fundraising performance.

But first, let's pull back the curtain for a closer look at Joseph's and Susan's situations.

With a staff of more than 20, Joseph experienced some difficulties in consistently meeting cost-per-dollar-raised targets, even before the economic turmoil at the end of the last decade. Now that the economy was on the mend, the upswing in fundraising he had anticipated wasn't happening. In fact, his multi-million, five-year campaign was stalled going into

14 Giving USA, accessed Feb. 23, 2014 at http://nonprofitquarterly.org/philanthropy/22476-giving-usa-2013-giving-coming-back-slowly-and-different-after-recess://ion.html
15 Ibid

year three of its silent phase. His reported cost per dollar raised last year was 50 cents. His board was beginning to ask uncomfortable questions.

A quick data check showed major gifts were responsible for less than one-third of Joseph's foundation's fundraising revenue. A subsequent rough calculation showed about 15% of total staff hours worked was focused on major gifts. Employees with principal responsibilities for major gifts (either front-line or support) numbered about 25% of the total staff, but a quick analysis of how those staff members actually spent their time revealed that each spent less than half of his time on major gifts. Time spent by the major gifts staff on special events, special projects, and administrative responsibilities actually exceeded time focused on major donors. Major gifts officers were averaging two or three donor-facing meetings a week.

Susan's situation was similar, though she was showing a better cost per dollar raised. Her fast-paced fundraising staff was saying grace over a myriad of projects—some of them contributing little to actual fundraising—with every staffer wearing many hats. The amount raised annually was up, though in constant dollars performance was flat compared to the years preceding the recession. She was proud of her very busy staff, but she worried about staff burnout.

Timesheet studies of both staffs found more time overall being spent on events than on any other category. The second largest time-spent category was annual gifts.

Finding a Way to Focus on Major Gifts

Willie Sutton, the last-century bank robber, is known, albeit apocryphally, for the urban legend that he answered a question about why he robbed banks with, "Because that's where the money is." There's a fundraising lesson here. Gail Perry, a well-known speaker and fundraising consultant, calls major gifts "every fundraiser's pot of gold."[16] That's where the money is.

---

16   Perry, Gail, How to Sabotage (or Save) Your Major Gift Program, accessed Feb. 23, 2014
     at http://www.gailperry.com/2010/11/how-to-sabotage-or-save-your-major gift-program/

Back in the corridor at the meeting, Joseph had shared his plan to "beef up" the staff by hiring a senior development executive. But, he also admitted, he hadn't moved on that plan because of a concern about making his current expense ratio even worse.

"It's a real dilemma," he said. "I desperately need somebody to get some of the day-to-day stuff off my plate and to take charge of the major gifts effort. But I just don't know how I will justify another staff position to my board."

"I can't cut somewhere else," he added. "Everybody is already maxed out with our workload."

Joseph's and Susan's dilemma is actually quite common. Many healthcare fundraising operations are *understaffed* relative to potential but *overstaffed* relative to current performance.

As Joseph suspected deep in his heart, simply adding staff can make the problem worse. A more systemic solution—one to address root cause issues—is needed.

Joseph recently had learned a little about Lean and Six Sigma in healthcare. He also remembered hospital in-service workshops that focused on quality initiatives with names like TQM and PDCA. But all of that had seemed much more relevant to clinical and patient experience functions than to a relationship-oriented discipline like fundraising. And the name *Lean* brought to mind unpleasant images of budget-cutting and staff reductions.

However, with health systems beginning to adopt Lean as a central transformation strategy, both Joseph and Susan were curious to learn if it might be an answer. And in this, they are like an increasing number of their peers. Whether the problem is a stalled campaign, deteriorating or flat year-to-year performance, or simply trying to cope with increased expectations for producing more from philanthropy, chief development officers and their healthcare system beneficiaries are increasingly willing to try new approaches.

The Power of Process

Performance improvement has a positive impact in fundraising just as in other areas. Process engineering, work-flow redesign, application of IT-supported measures, cycle-time metrics, and continuous improvement are as relevant to raising money as they are to higher patient satisfaction scores, improving ED throughput, and avoiding post-surgical readmissions.

Today, healthcare is embracing *process* as the key to quality, safety, and cost improvement. In fact, hospitals are beginning to adapt and embrace manufacturing quality principles, originally TQM[17] and more recently those employed in Toyota's Lean and GE's Six Sigma programs.

Applying Lean and Six Sigma to the people-intensive processes of patient care can prevent medical errors, decrease mortality rates, reduce lengths of stay, and increase patient and family satisfaction. Virginia Mason Medical Center, located in Seattle, Washington, and named multiple times a Top Hospital by The Leapfrog Group,[18] is known for applying Lean to improve quality and effectiveness in healthcare.

Virginia Mason also provided proof-of-concept for Lean in philanthropy by demonstrating dramatic fundraising improvement as the result of performance-improvement initiatives.[19]

A Lean organization strives to cut waste and increase value for customers by creating an efficient flow of products and services. Six Sigma is a disciplined, data-driven approach to eliminate defects in any process. When you combine the methodologies, Lean Six Sigma

---

17 Total Quality Management (TQM) is a system of organization-wide efforts to install and make permanent a climate in which an organization continuously improves its ability to deliver high-quality products and services to customers. TQM efforts typically draw heavily on the previously-developed tools and techniques of quality control. TQM enjoyed widespread attention during the late 1980s and early 1990s before being overshadowed by ISO 9000, Lean manufacturing, and Six Sigma.

18 The Leapfrog Group is a coalition of public and private purchasers of employee health coverage founded more than a decade ago to work for improvements in healthcare.

19 Jachim, Jeanne, Transforming the Major Gift Process, AHP International Conference, 2012.

emphasizes speed, reduced waste, and making the best use of staff and volunteer resources through a powerful data-driven system.

Performance-Improvement Imperatives

While Lean Six Sigma isn't rocket science, some performance improvement principles can be a bit counterintuitive. But once you start thinking in the way that working with Lean Six Sigma leads you, it seems to become common sense.

Many books have been written on the subject, so this chapter will neither attempt to teach Lean Six Sigma theory nor illustrate performance improvement tools. Instead, the focus will be on specific performance improvement applications in fundraising based on Lean Six Sigma principles.

Here are six imperatives in applying Lean Six Sigma principles to create fundraising processes that are more effective.

1. **Use high-cost, scarce resources to do only high-value work.** Good development officers are truly a scarce resource. For instance, they should focus on cultivating prospects, not on making database entries or other routine tasks. Can a clerical staffer input the data instead? What about things such as routine reporting, other paperwork, helping out with events, writing thank you letters and stewardship activities? What can you take off their plates to increase the number of true major gift prospect-facing meetings per week?

2. **Develop high-volume, point-of-entry activities and programs to create abundant prospect flow into the pipeline.** For example, in one model the initial *connector*, often a board member, brings people to interesting events where they learn about new initiatives or treatment advances. Some become qualified prospects and move through the process. A good metric is, for every

10 people brought in by the initial connector, one gives a gift at the target level (usually one or two more gifts at lesser levels also result). These *connects* are critical since staff people generally do not move in the social and business circles where potential major donors are found.

3. **Set critical-to-quality process measures, with emphasis on cycle time**. How many prospecting events will you hold each month? How many connections should you make at each event? How many prospects should you be cultivating at each stage? You must establish critical-to-quality (CTQ) criteria to let you know how you're doing, as well as a system for alerting you when a particular measure is or isn't being met. For example, you can use a dashboard system, where green means you're on track, yellow is the continuous-improvement zone, and red calls for immediate attention because you're seriously behind where you need to be.

4. **Measure early, measure often, and ensure your metrics have a causal relationship to success.** Instead of simply measuring things at the end, such as how much money was raised or the total sum each development officer brought in, use measures that help you see at key points whether you are on track for a positive outcome. Not only will you get what you measure, you will build a reliable forecasting system. Your CFO will love you. But beware metrics that may *correlate* with success but are not measuring those things that *cause* success.

5. **Maintain a constant effort to eliminate out-of-bounds process variance.** Create your "way" of fundraising, so you have a tried-and-true baseline process that is ingrained in your culture. In other words, if you have

four—or 14—gift officers, you will still have one consistent way your organization goes about acquiring gifts, instead of four to 14 different ways, with numerous variations from each. That one way should simultaneously allow for a clearly limited degree of variance and allow your front-line people to apply their experience and creativity to specific situations. You can then continuously improve that one way. (This is the Six Sigma aspect of the thinking.)

6. **Focus on high-return activities**. A basic principle of Lean is flexibly placing resources where they will generate the most value. One aspect of applying this principle is to focus sufficient resources on major gifts. Of course, you need a complete pyramid of fundraising strategies and methods, but if you focus on maximizing your major gifts program, you can significantly increase your ROI. A mark of a high-performing operation is a revenue mix of about 80% of total *dollars* coming from major gifts, which in number make up about 20% of total *gifts*.

Building Capacity

The Core Process[20] is a well-defined four-stage major- and middle-gift[21] process designed to qualify potential prospects, focus on those potential areas of support of most interest to the potential donor, build a relationship between the prospect and the beneficiary organization,

---

20 ©2006-2007, Marketing Partners, Inc. The term "Core Process" as applied to the fundraising process described and the graphic illustrations associated with it are protected by copyright. The Core Process was originally conceived by the author as a structure against which a training program could be applied. It quickly became apparent that the Core Process offered more than a theoretical basis for a training program.

21 Definitions of what level of contribution constitutes a major gift vary from to organization to organization. Some also use a "middle gift" definition for those contributions gained through the same or a similar face-to-face process as that involved with major gifts, but which are at a level lesser than major gifts.

and finally close the gift. It is named the "Core Process" because it is at the heart, or core, of the organization's fundraising effort—responsible for 80% or more of the total amount raised annually, if deployed correctly.

A key element is the application of stage-gate theory from the world of commercial product development. Stage gates are used in product development as a way of limiting investment risk by focusing on a progressively smaller and smaller number of the most promising new products as they move through development stages.

The three-stage textbook model for major gifts is *Identify-Cultivate-Solicit*. The core process became a four-stage model by separating *Engage* from the *Identify* and *Cultivate* stages, adding it as the second stage. The team-based "Tipping Point" concept–based on the work and research of author Malcolm Gladwell and shared in his bestselling book *The Tipping Point*[22]—is integrated into the process.

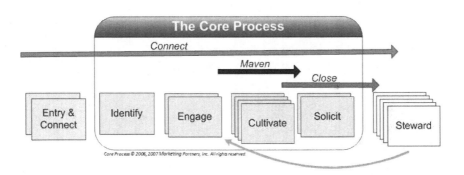

Identify

This is the stage immediately after the *connect*, in which a potential prospect is qualified as a prospect through one or two meetings with a development officer. It is a *listening* stage in which development officers guide the conversation in a way to enable them to assess the degree to which the potential prospect has the philanthropic capacity and inclination to be a significant donor.

---

22 Gladwell, M, The Tipping Point: How Little Things Can Make a Big Difference, Little Brown and Company, New York, 2000

Engage

If the prospect has demonstrated a propensity toward philanthropy, a sufficient affinity or link with the organization, and an interest in further exploration, the process moves to the *Engage* stage. It is here when the development officer begins to explore in depth with the prospect the various philanthropic opportunities that might match his, her, or their interests. This is the *focusing* stage. Development officers seek to understand which aspects of the case excite the prospect and with which level of giving a prospect is comfortable. If the prospects can be matched with an aspect of the case at an appropriate giving level, they are moved to the *Cultivate* stage.[23]

Cultivate

Once a match is found, the real romance begins as the potential donor is given significant exposure to the area in which he or she is interested as well as to the organization as a whole. This is the *relationship-building* stage. Development officers, campaign volunteers, and beneficiary executives work to ensure the prospect meets all the right people, becomes very well-informed about the philanthropic opportunity, and has the experiences that will solidify commitment to the cause. A positive response to a "trial ask"[24] will move the prospect to the *Solicit* stage.

---

23 Engage truly is a separate step from Identify. While the first stage was essentially a qualification of the prospects capacity for, and fundamental interest in philanthropy relative to the institution, Engage focuses attention on where the match might exist between donor interests and beneficiary needs.

24 Each of the Core Process stages involve an "ask." It is a permission-based, opt-in process. While the formal solicitation, which is often termed "the ask" in fundraising jargon, occurs in the fourth stage, the intent of the core process is to make solicitation a process, not a single event. Positive responses are stage-gate criteria for moving to the next stage. The "ask" in the first stage is for information regarding the potential prospect's interest in philanthropy through a discussion of why favorite charities are supported. In the second stage, the prospect is given an opportunity to agree to a "comfort level," which is a possible gift range in support of a specific philanthropic focus. The third stage's "trial ask," which in a sense is the real solicitation, "tests the water" by informally determining if the prospective donor will be comfortable with the specific formal solicitation planned for the next stage.

Solicit

This is the *closing* stage. The final step in the Core Process *begins* with the formal solicitation and continues through finalizing a gift agreement, recognition plan, and all of the many details that can be involved with receiving a major gift.

The Core Process combines the principles of fundraising relationship management with Lean Six Sigma thinking. The result is an ongoing process that focuses tightly on the key activities to shepherd a potential prospect from an initial contact through critical fundraising relationship management stages. It is designed for a team-based environment and provides an easily implemented step-by-step process through which the work of the development team is channeled and accelerated.

Measures and metrics are integral to the Core Process. They empower process-based management that, in turn, leads to employee engagement, which leads to increased organizational alignment and productivity. But it is true that "you get what you measure," so choose your measures carefully.

Sometimes even performance improvement professionals tend to ignore high-value measurements simply because they can be harder to measure. To correct for such measurement inversion, you must test your measures to ensure you focus on what is truly important. The ability to be precise in certain measures can be a siren song. Vaguely right is better than precisely wrong!

The application of metrics changes everything. And, that, of course, is a problem as well as the solution. People don't like change—and many aren't too wild about numbers, either. In fundraising, the objection sometimes is that all this somehow offends the essence of philanthropy, which is about authentic relationships and motivations for good.

Discussion of cycle time—the measurement of which is a core Lean principle—can result in a counterargument that fundraising is different than other processes. The stated objection may be that relationship building is, as it is so often put, "a marathon, not a sprint." Yet the time traditionally allotted for relationship-building in major gifts fundraising often involves longer spans than those typical in the development of personal or business relationships.

The reality is that speed matters. Not "hurry-up-and-ask" speed, but the kind of speed that comes from clarity of purpose, well-defined processes, active listening, intensity of effort, and continued focus on creating meaningful experiences for those prospects inclined to give.

Reaching Your Constituencies

The structure and composition of the healthcare fundraising board is critical to success in raising major gifts. Traditional thinking often results in a small, governance-oriented board with neither significant personal giving capacity nor the right connections. Often, such boards focus on oversight of fundraising rather than helping to raise funds themselves. And if the board doesn't lead the way, expecting others to volunteer to be part of the fundraising team is wishful thinking.

One of the biggest challenges fundraising executives face is getting board members, campaign volunteers, and institutional partners to help raise money. Getting beyond the *give and govern* role mentality typical of healthcare fundraising boards is difficult. What's missing is a specific role in a well-defined process that integrates board members and others into the fundraising team.

That role is one that Malcolm Gladwell terms the *Connector*. Board members and others use their personal and business connections to identify potential donors and facilitate introductions to them.[25]

This is a more narrowly defined, less time-intensive, but more valuable approach to volunteer involvement in fundraising. It is one with great appeal to those who don't want to attend a lot of meetings or be involved in asking for money. Individuals with personal giving capacity

---

25 The Tipping Point concept as applied to fundraising was originally created by Terry Newmyer, then Chief Development Officer at the Florida Hospital Foundation, Orlando.

and high-dollar connections can work as initial connectors in partnership with staff in a process-based major gifts model.

Without active participation of board members (and the involvement of other community- or constituency-based volunteers) as connectors, hospitals struggle to build major gift pipelines. Unlike higher education with its built-in potential donor pool of alumni, or other organizations with easily identifiable and reachable constituents, healthcare often must start from scratch to identify potential major donors within the community at large. Professional fundraising staff members rarely spend time in the same social or business circles as wealthy potential donors, but the members of a strong fundraising board do. Such board members, themselves committed leadership donors, can connect the development staff with high-potential prospects.

The *Tipping Point* concept was first applied, along with the Core Process, with extraordinary success, in a $100 million capital campaign that raised nearly 90% of its target through major gifts and reached its target 15 months ahead of schedule—all with an expense-to-revenue ratio well below the "gold standard" of 20 to 25%. This was an extraordinary accomplishment for an organization that was spending $2 million per year to raise $3 million not long before.

Making this powerful approach work depends on assigning roles as *Connectors*, *Mavens*, and *Closers*, loosely based on roles identified by Malcolm Gladwell in his book. The responsibilities of each team member are aligned with the strengths of each participating in the team-based fundraising effort.

Connectors—usually board members and campaign volunteers—are very much "people people." They identify prospects from their extensive collections of acquaintances and make the introductions that bring potential prospects into the process.

Mavens are the experts—often physicians and healthcare executives; sometimes board members or planned giving specialists—who offer credentials and provide knowledge that build prospect confidence in the organization and credibility for the case.

Closers—analogous to Gladwell's salesmen—are the transaction managers of the fundraising process. They are responsible for its culmination. Often the Closer role is filled by full-time development professionals, but volunteers, physicians, and healthcare executives who are oriented to asking for gifts can play a role too. Sometimes the *Closer* and formal *solicitor* roles are separated, with a board member, campaign volunteer, physician or executive asking for the gift. This does not diminish the role or real work of the Closer. The essence of the role is ensuring the right solicitation is made at the right time by the right person with the right materials, and that the necessary follow-through begins immediately to secure a pledge agreement.

Just focusing a process-improvement effort on major gifts will enable a significant increase in the amount raised—if done right. But sustained performance improvement that doubles or triples the amount raised annually does require a more comprehensive four-part approach.

The Other Pillars of High-Performance Fundraising

It would be a mistake to think process alone is enough. In order to yield the fullest ROI, the performance-improvement effort must focus on all four pillars of high-performance fundraising.

The beauty of performance improvement is that, done right, it focuses simultaneously on both top-line performance and bottom-line efficiency. A well-planned performance improvement initiative will address opportunities in all aspects of the fundraising operation.

In addition to *Capacity*—process-based, metric-measured operations that multiply the effectiveness of the people involved—and *Constituency*—an effective structure that brings the right composition of board members, campaign volunteers, and institutional and community partners to the fundraising process—two more pillars are essential: *Culture* and *Case*.

The first of these, *Culture*, is creating an organizational culture *for* philanthropy that recognizes the unique opportunities for, and requirements of, successful fundraising operations. The second, *Case*, involves developing a compelling, attention-getting, *donor-centric* reason to give, oriented to today's investor philanthropists.

Creating a Culture FOR Philanthropy

Much has been written about creating a *culture of philanthropy*. Unfortunately, the term appears often to be misunderstood, leading to initiatives focused on employee giving, elevating appreciation for the virtues of philanthropy, and recognizing the good things done in the community with charitable dollars—all of which are good, laudable, and worthwhile, but all of which miss the point.

Perhaps a better way of saying it would be to speak of creating a *culture for philanthropy*.

Edgar Schein, professor at the MIT Sloan School of Management, is one of many experts who say culture is the most difficult organizational attribute to change.[26] Charles Hill of the University of Washington and Gareth Jones of Texas A&M University define organizational culture as "the specific collection of values and norms shared by people and groups in an organization that controls the way they interact with each other and with stakeholders."[27]

In many cases, poor performance of the fundraising function reflects a Rodney Dangerfield "I don't get no respect" status within the health-care organization. And often that poor performance isn't recognized as such since expectations are low and there's no appetite on management's part to go out of its way to promote successful fundraising.

Reynold Levy, former president of New York's Lincoln Center and author of *Yours for the Asking*,[28] is one of many who believes the role of the CEO and other leaders in philanthropy is "simply indispensable." He notes that when setting out to raise a sum unprecedented for

---

26 Schein, E.H., Organizational Culture and Leadership, 3rd Ed., Jossey-Bass, San Francisco, 2010

27 Hill, C. L.; Jones, G. R., Strategic Management: An Integrated Approach, Sixth Edition, John Wiley & Sons, 2001

28 Levy, R., Yours for the Asking: An Indispensable Guide to Fundraising and Management, John Wiley & Sons, 2008

the organization, leadership must establish a culture for fundraising success.

Purposeful culture change comes from the top. The role of the CEO and the leadership team is not to be fundraisers themselves. It is to sponsor the function, ensuring adequate resources and a positive culture for philanthropy. Betsy Chapin Taylor, who coaches healthcare CEOs on building a culture for philanthropy, puts it this way, "The aim is not to create a swarm of solicitors but rather a chorus of believers."[29]

Creating a Breakthrough Case

A breakthrough case for support is one that dramatically differentiates the beneficiary institution in the marketplace in a way that makes achievement of significant performance-improvement targets possible.

Getting big gifts requires a big case for giving, something really exciting that can be tailored individually to the interests of large donors. The best way to get a major gift breakthrough case developed is as part of a process that partners with the health system—through a working partnership that reflects a positive culture for philanthropy—and includes input from the potential large donors. The beauty of such an approach is that for the same nickel it provides support to the case-development process while cultivating potential donors.

Relevance has always been essential to crafting an effective case for support. Michael VanDerhoef, president of the Virginia Mason Foundation, declared in 2008 the time had come in healthcare to change the case for support. Calling for more relevant and more ambitious non-traditional cases, he said, "We must fully appreciate the larger conversation that is already underway in our country, questioning the quality and cost of healthcare, and we must create a compelling message that defines philanthropic investment in healthcare as part of a larger solution."[30]

---

29 Taylor, B.C., Healthcare Philanthropy: Advance Charitable Giving to Your Organization's Mission, Health Administration Press, 2012.

30 Statement on AHP website accessed Feb. 22, 2014 at http://www.ahp.org/Home/Resources

Where do you start?

The goal is not to replace all other strategies with a major gift process. The end result should be a complete pyramid of fundraising strategies and methods (as well as an ongoing stewardship program), but one balanced between the *art* and *science* of fundraising in a way that maximizes return on the fundraising investment.

The *art* of fundraising embodies purposeful human interactions that build relationships and engender philanthropy. The *science* of fundraising uses accumulated knowledge acquired through disciplined empirical investigations in other settings and codified in systems such as Toyota's Lean to create more productive processes and flows. The first step in performance improvement is an assessment of the current program as the basis of a plan for change.

By these definitions, both art and science are needed to effectively elevate performance in healthcare fundraising. Hope isn't a strategy, but with an investment in performance improvement there *is* good reason for hope.

Executive Summary:

- Constraints to healthcare fundraising performance are primarily internal, not related to market potential. Many healthcare fundraising operations are *understaffed* relative to potential, even if some are *overstaffed* relative to current performance.
- The Four Pillars of Performance Improvement—as well as the *Connector*, *Maven*, and *Closer* team concept and a stage-gated major gifts process—are part of a new approach based on Lean Six Sigma thinking to improve healthcare fundraising performance. Today, healthcare

is embracing *process* as the key to quality, safety, and cost improvement. Performance improvement investments pay off in fundraising just as in other areas.

- Metrics are integral to harnessing the power of process. Process-based management leads to employee engagement, increased organizational alignment, and productivity. But "You get what you measure," so choosing measures carefully is vital. It would be a mistake to think process alone is enough.

- The performance improvement effort must focus on all four pillars of high-performance fundraising—*Capacity, Constituency, Culture*, and *Case*—focusing simultaneously on top-line performance and bottom-line efficiency.

Discussion

1. How does the author differentiate Lean and Six Sigma? How does he define the organizational result of combining the methodologies? How might that apply to healthcare fundraising?

2. The Four Pillars of Performance Improvement are *Capacity, Constituency, Culture*, and *Case*. What are the benefits of each?

3. Malcolm Gladwell's book *The Tipping Point* identifies *Connectors, Mavens, and Salesmen* as three necessary actors in social change. How does this chapter apply the concept in fundraising?

4. The chapter explores a four-part fundraising *Core Process,* which incorporates stage-gate concepts. How does this *Core Process* combine the principles of fundraising relationship management with Lean Six Sigma thinking?

5. In what ways are connectors, mavens, closers, measures and metrics integral to the Core Process?

Author Bio

Steven A. Reed is chairman of Marketing Partners, Inc., and president of its Performance Advantage subsidiary, which focuses on performance improvement in healthcare, including the application of Lean Six Sigma principles in healthcare fundraising. He is also a founding faculty member of the Fundraising Performance Institute.

Insights and Impacts of Benchmarking

Randy Varju, MBA, FAHP, CFRE

THERE IS A BENCHMARKING EXPERIMENT you can try the next time you present in front of an audience of 50 or more people. Mention that you want to make sure you are all on the same wavelength and that you'd like them to attempt to read your mind. Ask them first to think of the first color that comes to mind. It's important that they keep the first color and don't switch their choice. Then ask them to think of the first flower. Finally, ask them to think of the first piece of furniture. Now that they have their choices, ask them by a show of hands how many chose red as the color, rose as the flower, or couch as the piece of furniture. You may be as surprised as your audience by how many hands are raised. Chances are that, if they didn't pick all three, they will have at least selected one of them. But instead of some marvel of telepathy, what you really did is illustrate a simple exercise in benchmarking. If you don't like the questions I suggested, just find an old *Family Feud* game and pick the top responses to any three questions surveyed.

Benchmarking is a far more common part of our daily lives than we realize. How do you determine when your car needs gas? What was your GPA in high school? What resumes will get past the first round for that position you're looking to fill? We are constantly gathering information, interpreting data, and making decisions based on how this information compares to thresholds or norms.

When considering benchmarking as a development tool, most jump right to the thought of lengthy surveys, dread of tedious data pulls, and worry of how they will rank. Instead, the focus should be on determining areas for priority impact, assessments that shape resource allocation, and tolerance for performance variability. This then pivots benchmarking from a one-time data dump to an ongoing driver for a culture of heightened performance with impact.

In healthcare, little happens without measuring, tracking, and benchmarking. The process of navigating symptoms leading to a diagnosis and prescribed treatment offers a well-established pathway to consistent, predictable outcomes. Our ability to track and share data allows us to communicate with others on familiar terms. It builds credibility and understanding with caregivers, volunteers, executive leaders, and donors. It broadens their appreciation for the important measures in philanthropy and connects our efforts to the other successes of the organization.

Stepping on the Scale

Getting started requires a careful consideration of the resources available and required for your organization. It starts by looking inside instead of out. If you're in a smaller institution, you will need to confirm that your practices and definitions are consistent with those you intend to compare your organization against. The Association for Healthcare Philanthropy (AHP) offers a *Standards Manual* that provides clear definitions for the most helpful industry practices. If you're in a larger shop or a in a healthcare system, you will need to make sure your practices and definitions are not only consistent with the comparison pool but also consistent within the various components of your institution. This is a growing challenge as systems integrate new hospitals and look to incorporate their data as well. Calibrating reporting expectations and procedures is frequently necessary to assure each team member is working from a common set of reporting definitions. This also includes establishing a culture of individual accountability. It is not just the foundation as a whole that is affected by benchmarking. The collective effort of each team member is essential in shifting your overall performance. Understandably, measuring staff resources and productivity can create anxiety for some. Your team must collectively embrace and commit to an environment motivated and driven by high performance. Tracking individual performance then serves as a means of identifying efficiencies, aggregating and removing barriers to heightened performance, and rewarding achievements.

Defining what you hope to accomplish on the front end will also help you gather the resources you will need to guide you in preparing your institution. Clarity of purpose will unite solid teams in collective effort. But you can't determine where you are headed until you assess where you are starting. Ultimately, there is no substitute for stepping on the scale in helping to determine how much work you have to do. Weighing in as a team and as members of a team sets the baseline. In order to set goals and eventually celebrate progress, those who are critical to driving results must fully understand the current state and the role they play in achieving improvements. But before jumping in to a comprehensive benchmarking study, there are a number of internal functional assessments you can make that will help determine your priority focus areas and critical deliverables.

A good place to start is with longstanding resources that will help you compare your current baseline. *Giving USA: The Annual Report on Philanthropy* is one such resource. This publication estimates total sources and uses of charitable giving in the United States each year, utilizing well-established methodologies. The most recent information reported can be found by visiting givingusareports.org. One of the many helpful graphics the report offers is a breakdown of giving by source of contributions. A simple comparison to your current donor mix offers valuable insights and can serve as a good starting point to your top-line assessment. The graphic uses four categories to report giving by source: individuals, foundations, bequests, and corporations.

If you annually review data as part of your reporting to volunteer leaders, you likely have a similar graphic that illustrates your own donor mix. While this information is for philanthropy as a whole, AHP also provides a similar breakdown for the funds that are specifically reported by healthcare institutions, with a few additional categories. Comparing your information to nationally benchmarked results not only begins to establish credibility for your efforts but also will uncover some insights to guide longer-term foundational strategies for your leadership team.

For instance, let's start with corporations. In the most recent study available at the time of this writing, corporations contributed $18.15 billion, or 6% of total philanthropy for that year.[31] If you incorporate the broader definition of Business & Corporation Foundations, as measured by AHP, the percentage grows to 17% specifically for healthcare institutions submitting data.[32] After reviewing the definitions of either of these comparison points, you can pull the corresponding data for your institution. Is your proportion of corporate giving higher or lower than the percentages reported for either of these studies? If it is significantly lower, this may offer an opportunity for focus to determine if there are further efforts that would elevate your outcomes. If, instead, your numbers are similar or higher, it shows you are either maximizing your efforts in this area or you are in a corporate corridor where these gifts are a larger portion of your portfolio. This simple comparison also offers valuable insight for your volunteer and executive leadership. It is common for these groups to assume there is far greater opportunity for fundraising in the corporate sector than the national or healthcare-specific averages illustrate. If you can show your efforts are in alignment with industry ratios, you can make a stronger case for focusing efforts on other sections of the donor mix. Ultimately you can allocate more time, energy, and resources to securing more corporate gifts. But

---

31 Giving USA Foundation, Giving USA: The Annual Report on Philanthropy (Indiana University Lilly Family School of Philanthropy, 2013), 2012 Contributions by source of contributions.

32 The Association for Health Care Philanthropy, AHP Performance Benchmarking Service General Overview Report, (The Associate for Health Care Philanthropy, 2012), Constituency Giving, overall percent of combined production.

if you are already performing at or above the nationally benchmarked levels, you are not likely to see results that significantly exceed either of these percentage outcomes, regardless of the effort allocated.

Continue this comparison with each segment of your current donor mix. You will determine what sets you apart from other institutions, and more importantly, what priority areas offer potential for your most significant growth. Admittedly this is a very basic assessment. But it gives you a place to start as well as a well-recognized national resource to back your findings in establishing the value of benchmarking. It will also help shape conversations with your leadership team around opportunities that exist. This is just the first layer of your assessment. Before you can start shifting resources or determining what metrics you want to track or what goals you want to achieve, you will need to compare what you know about your donor mix with the existing culture and landscape of the institution you serve.

It probably hasn't been too long since you've walked through a nursing or telemetry unit in your hospital. The continuous monitoring of patients allows care providers to respond quickly if complications arise. Through a set of vital signs, they are able to assess each patient and prescribe treatments as necessary.

If you were to assess your institution's philanthropic culture, you would likely arrive at a number of components that collectively represent and largely impact your ability to raise funds. Your ability to function and thrive is dependent on the mix of these variables. When strategically assessed in combination with the previous review of your donor mix, the profile of your foundation's landscape starts to more clearly take shape. A simple ranking of these variables can be a helpful exercise for your team, your executive leadership, and your lead volunteers (see Philanthropy Vital Signs, below). Once again, using corporate giving potential as an example, let's suppose you identify an opportunity for growth as a result of assessing your market profile and current donor mix. If you don't also score strengths in institutional funding opportunities, volunteer engagement, or executive leadership involvement, you will not likely maximize your potential breakthrough. Volunteer networking with corporate leaders, executive leadership that is willing to join on visits, and a healthy array of funding opportunities that align with corporate funding priorities all contribute significantly to the outcomes you can expect.

Philanthropy Vital Signs

	Strength	Neutral	Challenge
Market readiness (image/profile/market share)			
Array of funding opportunities			
Annual philanthropic track record			
Existing major gift portfolio			
Volunteer engagement			
Physician (care-giver) philanthropic partnerships			
Executive leadership/ involvement			

For multi-site systems, these variables will fluctuate based on the history, philanthropic maturity, or culture of each site. Monitoring these components will help you determine what priorities for internal improvement need to be addressed or which early opportunities can be leveraged regardless of the size of your institution. Likewise, for you to benefit from a focused effort in benchmarking, knowing where and how you will need to focus your efforts, apply your findings, and transform practices is critical. This exercise not only gives you a sense of how you can tailor benchmarking efforts to specific situations and preferred outcomes but also begins to broaden the collective understanding of the important role others play in the ultimate success of your institution's philanthropic efforts. If you do an associate giving campaign, how would you rate its current success? Is it a reflection of your institution's associate engagement or, more likely, a result of how the campaign is run? Do you compare year-to-year results in benchmarking each year's success? Likewise, do you track giving from your governance volunteers as a reflection of their dedication to your institution's mission? Do they give because they are asked or because they see the impact? When you begin to drive these connections, benchmarking becomes far more than tracking and sharing numbers. It becomes a vehicle for driving philanthropic culture, maturity, and valuable linkages to your shared impact.

Comparison Points

Once you commit to comparing your organization to others, the options are plentiful. Benchmarking information is more accessible now than in any previous time in the fundraising profession. Data is abundant through numerous formal and informal channels. There are libraries of accumulated resources through the more prominent fundraising associations. There are countless online catalogs of data, articles, and presentations on the topic. Colleagues can join online groups, share information, and pose questions through numerous channels that simply didn't exist a few years ago. Depending on the specific issues you'd like to address or the type of information you'd like to gather, there are likely a number of other *similar* institutions you can find with a little effort and networking. Notice, though, the choice of the word *similar*. Some organizations spend a great deal of time fretting over finding the perfect match. However, development shops are like snowflakes: no two are exactly alike. Much of what organizations can gain from each other is found in similarities despite the many differences.

An example of this can be seen in the world of extreme sports. While watching the X Games BMX bike competition, you might gasp at the tricks performed. Somehow competitors jump a hill and do a backflip or even leave the bike, with only one hand on the seat. Interestingly, if you then watch the motocross competition, you'll see the same tricks on motorcycles. If that's not enough, you can then also see very similar tricks in the Winter X Games on snowmobiles. There is a good deal of difference between BMX bikes and snowmobiles. Yet, somehow, these young athletes have found a way to learn from each other by focusing on what they have in common. In turn, they each improve and astound.

While each of the emerging resources available today provides value in new and unique ways, there is still no substitute for participating in a well-established benchmarking study. While more formal and scientific, the challenge of finding the perfect cohort still exists. However, the more prominent studies have a well-tested means of removing much of the typical practice variance. While daunting and time-consuming, these studies offer findings that make the effort well worthwhile. The data-gathering process alone is an effective test of your capabilities and practices. You will find that after completing your first successful submission, you will benefit from more clearly defined protocols, practices, and standards within your team. The rigor in coordinating and preparing your team's data is likely to uncover areas of performance variability. This is an opportunity not to be overlooked in calibrating data-entry expectations and practices. Setting your standards at this stage will be valuable later when benchmarking reaches the individual level.

Allocating appropriate resources is also critical when participating in these more robust studies. You will likely find data analysis to be an area of interest or expertise for someone on your team. Enlisting that person in coordinating your efforts, gathering the data, interpreting the findings, and sharing the results will significantly improve the quality of your results. It will be a valuable experience for the team member and a tremendously helpful resource for your team. Assigning or finding your data specialist helps in consolidating your data with a singular, consistent perspective. In multi-hospital systems, pulling data from each of the individual sites can result in varied responses, based on their practice or interpretation of the survey tool. Having one person or a small team driving this process sets the uniform definitions in place and provides for the necessary consistency in reporting.

Participating in benchmarking is a commitment, so carefully consider the content deliverables of each option and how these deliverables align with the intended uses of the information. The AHP Performance Benchmarking Service, for instance, allows participants to compare data in a number of valuable ways while also using a time-tested set of definitions that remove much of the reporting variability from participants. In addition to a program review using return on investment (ROI) as a means of ranking, there are more detailed program-level analyses for major giving, planned giving, annual giving, special events, and public support. Within each of these areas, participants receive data focusing on their net production revenue, fundraising expenses, ROI, and cost to raise a dollar. Coupled with the participant data and comparative placements in the study's ranges, there is valuable narrative that highlights a number of performance factors, trends, and conclusions that can help further guide individual takeaways.

Regardless of the benchmarking tool you select, it is likely to use ROI as a significant comparison point. Be aware that ROI is a familiar measure in numerous fields and, at times, can be considered a pivotal determinant in perceived success or failure. Use care in crafting an understanding of ROI as a measure of efficiency. This can be done by building an understanding of the ROI norms for the practices in your donor mix. When combined with other critical criteria, it helps determine focal points for your efforts, but it shouldn't be the only determinant for an effort's survival. While events and direct mail are more costly and, in turn, have a lower ROI, they provide value that doesn't turn up in the numbers. They broaden your networking reach and replenish your prospect portfolio in ways that shouldn't be dismissed. However, if your efforts are clearly underperforming based on the benchmarked ranges, there is cause to scrutinize your current practice. Likewise, if you are primarily dependent on events, annual fund, or grants, ROI numbers coupled with benchmarked individual gift deliverables can help you build a solid case for developing and driving a major gifts effort.

The true success in benchmarking is not in looking at the survey and celebrating those areas where you outrank your peers. Sure, it's tempting. But that misses the point. Instead it is in interpreting the findings in a manner that will help guide your strategies and improve your outcomes. To effectively accomplish this, the process should be embraced as a means of comparing yourself to what is intended as an industry composite of similar entities. This in combination with your donor mix and vital signs assessment from earlier will help identify a few key focus areas unique to your environment and culture.

The Vital Few

It's hard not to be overwhelmed with the amount of data returned after a formal benchmarking study. There's a tendency to want to read it all, digest it quickly, and set about all of the plans necessary to improve everything at once. Keep in mind, most prescriptions have a pacing and dosage warning that comes with the directions. Carefully think of your implementation plans in much the same way. Keep to the "two aspirin every four hours" strategy for maximum benefit. Also be careful to assess each of the variables based on their priority and impact. Not all data points will apply as urgently or directly as others. Those that truly matter stand out as part of your personal profile for improvement.

A relatable concept is participating in a NASCAR driving experience. You suit up and climb into one of the cars you've seen on occasion driving nearly 200 miles per hour on TV. You would likely be surprised by how unfamiliar it is. The helmet is tight, there is very little room, and you can't turn your head at all to check any blind spots. Fortunately, there are spotters who communicate through earpieces wedged in the helmet to guide you through each step. Naturally, you would look around for anything familiar—only to realize there is no speedometer. The gauges include water temperature, water pressure, oil temperature, oil pressure, and one larger gauge for RPMs, but there is no speedometer. That's because the dashboard has room for only those items most essential to the car's performance. Speed is irrelevant in this case as long as you're a bit faster than the car behind you. Honestly, knowing the speed would be a distraction with all of the information you are already processing in such an unfamiliar setting. It might even work against you by serving as motivation to push for some threshold speed you aren't skilled to safely manage.

Determining the key metrics that will populate your dashboard is a valuable step in shaping the activities that lead to improved results. Beyond the dashboard, there are other measures you may define as spotters, those that determine pacing and course corrections along the way. You may even identify your network of professional colleagues as spotters in a way. There are things they can likely see from the stands that you can't see from behind the wheel. Regardless of the type or size of your shop, the benchmarking process builds from a set of experiences, findings, and insights that ultimately drive discoveries unique to your culture and philanthropic life-stage. Translating the accumulation of these insights into actionable priorities can require some heavy sifting. Revisit your original intent in considering benchmarking. Was it to determine your greatest opportunity for growth? Was it to justify new staff positions in major gifts? Was it to broaden your efforts beyond annual fund, grants, and special events? Given the unique variables of your environment, the process outlined to this point should provide a framework for guiding your vision and goals. It should provide ample backing in sound industry practice to validate your recommendations. It should enhance volunteer and executive engagement in strategic efforts aligned to mutually advance support of your institution. Carrying out that vision now transitions from data collection and interpretation to individual practice and accountability.

"Pulling" Your Weight

In the book *The Power of Pull*,[33] the authors underscore the importance of attracting like-minded people in fully leveraging sources of knowledge and passion. It is through the people you attract (or pull) that you can make the transition from the information you gather to the knowledge you apply.[34] The authors also use the fitting term *Return on Attention* to underscore the power of collective effort and knowledge focused on key outcomes.[35] In healthcare, a comparison can be found in the many safety efforts that require both individual and collective attention. The return in this case is a safe environment for every patient. This isn't achieved easily. But by enlisting experts from the airlines and nuclear industry, healthcare institutions are undergoing a transformation with aspirations of eliminating any and all harm of patients. One of the ways this attention is focused is with daily huddles where each department reports on high-risk patients and provides a review of any issues or near misses. This persistent attention underscores the importance of the effort and addresses any variance in real-time. If you have participated in one of these meetings, you likely came away amazed at how much can be covered and accomplished in the span of a 15- to 20-minute meeting. Much can be gained in applying this same rigor to your team and individual development efforts. Finding the right focal points for this attention is vital to delivering intended outcomes.

There are a number of industry standard metrics that help track the accountabilities of development professionals regardless of the role they serve. By limiting the focus to a vital few that populate each dashboard, there is an obvious and intentional priority, or attention, allocated to those efforts necessary to drive heightened performance in the areas you determine most crucial. While you can't control every variable that potentially impacts your ability to raise funds, you can manage those

---

33 John Hagel III, John Seely Brown, Lang Davison, The Power of Pull: How Small Moves, Smartly Made, Can Set Big Things in Motion (New York: Basic Books, 2010), 173.

34 Hagel, Brown, Davison, The Power of Pull, 174.

35 Hagel, Brown, Davison, The Power of Pull, 172.

efforts and activities that maximize your potential to do so. When determining your set of metrics or dashboard gauges, be sensitive to the necessary balance of both outcome and activity goals. Additionally, while outcome goals like dollars-raised or activity goals like solicitations-made address current production expectations, there is an ongoing need to provide for longer-term production capacity. Determine the most valuable measurements you can implement to assure proper portfolio replenishment. Also, if you are in a larger system with numerous sites or service-line structures, it will be important to reflect both work-unit as well as system-level goals.

There is a careful balance between driving, focusing, and reviewing the numbers versus forming deeper, valuable, meaningful relationships with donors and prospects. Some will feel an overemphasis on the numbers can take away or somehow diminish the true intent of individual relationship-building. What data has shown, however, is that these two deliverables are not exclusive of one another. Being intentional and strategic with your daily or weekly priorities instead allows you to build and track more relationships. High-performing gift officers consistently manage the metrics while in no way diminishing the genuine nature of each donor interaction.

Aligning goals from the top down will also provide needed clarity for each team member regarding the priorities placed on each objective. This should connect all the way to the performance-review process. This provides for consistent feedback tailored for each individual and each role. Obviously, once a year at performance-review time doesn't give you an opportunity for timely course corrections, though. There are tools that help share status updates daily, weekly, or monthly. These range from visual tracking boards or electronic reports to team meetings. Regardless, there is a natural reluctance to reporting and sharing individual data in an open team setting. Yet if you want to see immediate and consistent results in a specific area, there is no substitute. The key to gaining comfort is in rewarding the positives while tracking and removing the barriers to performance variance.

Borrowing from the Safety Huddle template, the Foundation for

Advocate Health Care, with 11 hospitals throughout Illinois, has had success with a half-hour Wednesday morning "Hump-Day Huddle" meeting by phone conference. The focus of the meeting is devoted to need-to-know topics for the week as well as brief reports from each team or department on their key metrics. Each leader reports for three to five minutes. Participants also look along on their desktops at a couple of key graphics that visually track the organization's progress. If the numbers are off track for any team, they provide a brief explanation or share the barriers they are facing. These variances are not only tracked but also reviewed once a month to look for common trends that require root-cause attention. These brief, weekly check-in calls also provide value beyond the positive impact they have clearly had on the metrics that are tracked by engaging the entire team as spotters in sharing the information necessary to keep collective efforts on track.

Where You Stand Versus How You Run

Whether at the macro level of nonprofit philanthropy or the micro level of individual performance, benchmarking starts with a motivation to improve. It is pushed by an appetite for consistent and sustainable results. In his book *How the Mighty Fall*, Jim Collins outlines some of the perils that lead to decline. One that relates to benchmarking is when "leaders discount negative data, amplify positive data, and put a spin on ambiguous data."[36] This is in contrast to the disciplined, open, and honest application of findings intended to transform your institution. It requires stamina to perform at your best.

When running a 5K or a marathon, you don't just show up expecting it to go well. You plan, prepare, and practice. Once you build up your endurance, you start tracking your best times. On race day, you get lined up, knowing you are prepared to finish, and you have a sense of your aspired and likely outcomes. Hopefully, you know your pace

---

36 Jim Collins, *How the Mighty Fall, and Why Some Companies Never Give In* (New York: HarperCollins, 2009), 22.

well enough to gauge how much is enough and when it is too much. Finishing the race is both exhilarating and rewarding, but the first thing most of us will do is look at our stopwatch. Did I beat my personal best? Sure, you may visit the result boards to see where you ended up in your age bracket, but the real determinant of success is how you did in relation to your own best time. If done well, benchmarking is about maximizing *your* performance to *your* capacity. The data points along the way help build a better understanding of that capacity based on what others similar to you have been able to accomplish and, thankfully, are open to sharing.

Executive Summary

- Benchmarking drives and requires a culture dedicated to heightened performance.
- Our ability to track and share data allows us to communicate with others on familiar terms and should be used in building a culture of shared philanthropic impact.
- No benchmarking cohort will be a perfect match. There is much to be gained by focusing on similarities and practices.
- Benchmarking is not about your institution's ranking. It is about continuously interpreting the findings in a manner that will help guide your strategies and improve your outcomes.
- Benchmarking is helpful at the institutional and individual level in focusing consistent rigor and collective effort.
- Benchmarking is meant to maximize **your** performance to **your** full capacity.

Discussion

1. Where do you see your best potential for growth?
2. What parts of your philanthropic culture need to advance before you can fully leverage the benchmarking process and resulting data?
3. How is philanthropy viewed within your institution? How could exposing key partners to strategies backed by benchmarking data work to your advantage?
4. What is your team tolerance for openly sharing data and performance? If there is reluctance, why?

Author Bio

Randy Varju, MBA, FAHP, CFRE, is president of the Advocate Charitable Foundation and chief development officer for Advocate Health Care. In this capacity, he has executive responsibility for the vision, planning, implementation, and management of charitable giving and fundraising for all Advocate hospitals and system-wide development initiatives. Advocate Health Care is the largest fully integrated healthcare delivery system in Illinois, with 1.1 million patients annually. It has been named one of the nation's top health systems based on clinical performance, according to Thomson Reuters. Varju serves on the Board of the Association of Health Care Philanthropy for North America as well as the Association of Fundraising Professionals, Chicago Chapter.

Key Partnerships for Success

CEOs Provide Critical Leverage
Betsy Chapin Taylor, FAHP

THE INVOLVED chief executive officer (CEO) is essential to achieve healthcare philanthropy's true potential. Healthcare philanthropy has emerged as a vital, next-curve revenue resource with the power to ensure sustainability or to capture competitive advantage. Since the healthcare CEO is entrusted with the successful management and financial health of the organization, this means his involvement in advancing philanthropy as a lever to organizational excellence is no longer optional. The CEO is uniquely positioned to convey his vision for the future, to give donors confidence, to provide critical internal support, to drive a culture for philanthropy, and to rally the meaningful engagement of key organizational advocates including boards and physicians.

The Burning Platform

The financial landscape for healthcare is littered with stumbling blocks.

- CEOs identify financial challenges as their top management concern.[37]
- More than 400 US hospitals have closed in the last two decades.[38]

---

37 "Top Issues Confronting Hospitals 2013", Healthcare Executive, March/April 2014, p. 88

38 "The Future of Hospitals in America", Richard J. Umbdenstock, Healthcare Executive, March/April 2014, p. 78

- One-third of US hospitals have a negative total operating margin.[39]
- By 2020, 20% of US hospitals are predicted to seek a merger partner.[40]

Lack of dollars to reinvest in the healthcare organization has become a common constraint. Financial scarcity stems from a variety of inter-related challenges including increasing operating costs, technological innovation, evolving standards of care, and the cost of physician recruit-ment. However, there is also ambiguity about the financial implications of health reform and its cornerstone piece of legislation: the Affordable Care Act (ACA). While this watershed legislation increases access to health insurance, it also triggers simultaneous and significant cuts to Medicare and Medicaid reimbursements and changes the formula for how hospitals are paid from a fee-for-service "volume" model to an amount-per-condition "value" model.

Clear financial risk for the foreseeable future makes the rationale for the healthcare CEO to embrace philanthropy simple: healthcare orga-nizations must find new and more effective ways to generate revenue to fuel growth and progress. Since philanthropy has demonstrated viabil-ity as a revenue resource with a rate of return that exceeds that of most clinical service lines, it is time for healthcare CEOs to take a proactive approach to positioning philanthropy as a core strategy and business strength to provide operational and capital dollars for organizational advancement. Having a high-performing philanthropy program has also become another valued sign of financial fitness; ratings agencies list the existence of a successful philanthropy program as an attribute of a sound healthcare organization.

---

39 AHA Trendwatch Chartbook 2013, August 27, 2013, http://www.aha.org/research/reports/tw/chartbook/2013/13chartbook-full.pdf

40 "New Laws and Rising Costs Create a Surge of Supersizing Hospitals", The New York Times, Julie Creswell and Reed Abelson, August 12, 2013

The CEO Quick List: 33 Ways for CEOs to Advance Philanthropy

Drive Culture:

- Communicate the organizational importance of philanthropy
- Embrace the healthcare organization as a charitable endeavor
- Establish giving as a whole-organization goal
- Create a process to ensure strategic alignment of funding priorities
- Ensure investment in development to enable capacity and growth
- Foster synergy between development, marketing, and PR
- Support collaboration between development and clinical operations
- Serve as a role model both as a donor and in donor cultivation
- Educate, engage, and mobilize healthcare executives and staff
- Include giving metrics on organizational dashboards/scorecards/goals
- Celebrate key gifts and donors from the boardroom to the front line
- Ensure visible symbols of the role and impact of giving in the facility

Leverage Allies:

- Actively seek the engagement of governing boards and physicians
- Set expectations for individual and collective board participation
- Ensure philanthropy is part of board and physician orientation
- Publicly affirm the positive impact of board and physician participation

- Routinely include philanthropy on key organizational agendas
- Help recruit specific advocates to specific high-value endeavors

Foster Relationships:

- Articulate the organization's compelling vision to donors/prospects
- Nurture authentic relationships with key donors/prospects
- Assist in donor cultivation, solicitation, and stewardship
- Attend key functions and meetings that advance philanthropy
- Communicate the hospital is a nonprofit, community-benefit organization
- Put donors first when "low value," avoidable calendar conflicts arise

Support Development:

- Make time for personal involvement in fund development roles
- Ensure access to organizational information, strategy and plans
- Position the CDO and development function for credibility inside and out
- Position the foundation/development office as the only way to give
- Facilitate HIPAA-approved access to patient information
- Use appropriate, predictive metrics to measure development
- Come to board meetings on time and without being attached to a phone
- Meet with the CDO one-on-one, regularly
- Make a personal financial gift commensurate with interest and ability

The Leadership Iceberg

Much attention is focused on the CEO's external roles in advancing philanthropy. Certainly, donors making significant, investment-level gifts expect to have not only an audience but also a relationship with the CEO. That's because the CEO is best positioned to espouse the organization's vision and to provide assurance of the organization's commitment and ability to execute on plans. However, the CEO's donor-facing role is the proverbial "tip of the iceberg": it is a visible symbol of involvement, but the bulk and greatest strength of the CEO in advancing philanthropy is hidden within the walls of the healthcare organization.

The symbolic and tactical importance of the CEO in prioritizing philanthropy within the organization cannot be overstated. No other organizational leader has the stature and relationships to single-hand-edly deploy the organization to advance philanthropy—or not. The CEO uses her verbal support, physical presence, and active modeling to signal that philanthropy is important, to elevate it on the agenda, to set expectations, to unleash resources, and to build momentum with advocates.

While there is a laundry list of strategic, cultural, and tactical opportunities for the CEO in advancing philanthropy, some of the most leveraged internal roles include:

- Positioning fund development as a strategic endeavor,
- Weaving philanthropy into the consciousness and com-mitment of employees, and
- Fostering the engagement of board members and physicians.

Alignment Drives Impact

CEOs can ensure tight alignment between the strategic priorities of the healthcare organization and the funding priorities of the fund develop-ment organization.

Many organizations squander the impact of philanthropy by allowing charitable dollars to benefit low-value activities and initiatives. This most often occurs when healthcare organizations fund items that rank highest during a capital or budget-planning process; then they give items left on the chopping block to the fund development organization. However, it is important to harness the power of philanthropy by ensuring it is directed toward high-value initiatives that are tightly aligned with the organization's highest strategic aspirations. Assurance that donor dollars will have a genuine impact is essential to attract major donors, who are inclined to direct their most significant giving toward high-impact, high-visibility projects that are central to the hospital's strategic plan and core mission.

To enable strategically aligned project selection, CEOs are encouraged to insist upon a clear, formal, diligent, and collaborative process to identify appropriate projects. Characteristics of qualified projects include:

- Consistency with the mission of the organization;
- Strategic importance to fueling progress, innovation, capacity, mission, or other objectives to achieve the organization's vision and potential;
- Additive value that will raise the standard of care rather than fulfilling basic business obligations including mandates, infrastructure, or replacements;
- Emotional appeal to donors by virtue of providing direct physical, emotional, or social benefits to patients and families;
- Time horizon to allow for donor identification, cultivation, and solicitation;
- Physician to champion the clinical value of the proposed solution; and
- Financial goal size that is achievable, meaningful, and based upon the availability and capacity of likely donors rather than simply representing the gap between dollars the organization has and dollars the organization needs.

An effective process would also include mechanisms to seek input and collaboration from executives, governing board members, foundation board members, and others with information that must be factored into a well-designed decision-making process. Projects selected through this process would then generally be taken to the entire foundation board for their consideration and input, since foundation leadership volunteers spearheading solicitation need to have input and ownership of funding priorities that will be presented to prospective donors.

CEO insistence on diligence in this most basic—but often poorly executed—task moves philanthropy from the realm of the decorative to the realm of the strategic.

Employees Enable Connectivity

Healthcare organization employees bring the connectivity of consistent—and often intense and personal—connections with patients and families, so employees must be enlisted as proponents for philanthropy. As the organization's highest-ranking leader, the CEO's words, efforts, and actions are essential to weave philanthropy into the everyday life of the employees who make up the organization. As the CEO frames how philanthropy impacts the organization's work, his endorsements and expectations set a standard that motivates employees to view the organization's nonprofit status as an essential part of its identity, to integrate philanthropy into their communications and language, to allocate time and attention, and to translate goals into specific process or behavioral changes.

Several conditions must exist to drive employee engagement in philanthropy:

- Everyone must understand how philanthropy makes a difference that impacts each member of the organization and those they serve.
- People must be passionate enough about their work to expand their vision of their own role beyond completing the task they are assigned (*e.g.*, being a nurse or providing

housekeeping) to fulfilling the overarching purpose of the organization (*e.g.*, providing hope and healing).

- Philanthropy must be linked back to the vision and values of the organization to weave it into the language, behaviors, norms, expectations, and rewards that make up "the way things get done around here."

There is a common objection from clinical caregivers the CEO can help overcome either directly or by engaging her own leadership team. For example, there will obviously be certain individuals with whom the foundation will want to interact during a patient care experience. Many organizations now take the opportunity to express gratitude, to make connections, or to elevate the level of service for current or prospective donors during an inpatient stay or outpatient visit. These activities to interact with and elevate service for select patients set off the silent alarm bells for many frontline staff members who balk at a perceived two-tiered care system. Therefore, assurances need to be made that these efforts do not impact the healthcare organization's commitment to provide the same high quality clinical care to all who come, regardless of ability to pay. Rather, this is an opportunity to strengthen relationships with current and potential partners. There is also value to explaining how the support of these particular patients positively impacts all who are served.

CEOs can help build an organizational culture for philanthropy when they ACT:

A: advocate for philanthropy as a strategic, mission-aligned endeavor,

C: connect giving to daily life by showing its relevance for everyone's work, and

T: tell stories to illustrate how philanthropy touches and saves lives.

Through the efforts of the CEO, his executives, and their managers, a commitment to philanthropy can cascade through the organization to not only add additional purpose to the work but also to ensure everyone is informed and prepared to express the value and opportunity of philanthropy.

Enfranchise Key Influencers

One of the most optimized roles for CEOs is broadening the base of leadership by engaging board members and physicians in philanthropy.

CEOs play a powerful gatekeeper role when it comes to accessing key advocates; because of the vital importance of relationships with boards and physicians, they may be buffered from efforts seen to be ancillary. The stature of the CEO as the visible head of the organization also gives her rare influence and gravitas to communicate priorities and to mobilize key parties. For these complementary reasons of opening access, elevating prioritization, and facilitating involvement, it is critical for the CEO to unlock the potential of key advocates.

Engage the Boards

Governing board and foundation board engagement provides a key performance advantage in advancing philanthropy. Both governing board and foundation board members open up crucial networks, provide leadership for philanthropic effforts, marshal various forms of internal and cultural support, and validate the importance of the healthcare mission to a larger public.

It is nearly impossible to gain access to the governing board without CEO endorsement. The CEO generally has the most trusted and substantive relationship with the healthcare organization's governing board, which makes her the best person to explain the rationale for philanthropy and to seek its engagement in this aspect of providing sound governance. The CEO has unparalleled power to set and encourage expectations for board member involvement in philanthropy, to place philanthropy on the orientation and training agenda, and to position philanthropy as a strategic endeavor of the healthcare organization that merits investment and attention. Ultimately, the governing board will not be fully engaged and empowered without the CEO serving as a catalyst.

The CEO also undeniably sets a tone for the relationship between the healthcare organization and foundation board. There are countless examples of CEOs carefully holding the foundation board at arm's length from the healthcare organization with the justification that foundation board members often serve a separate but related corporation. However, positioning the foundation board as a subordinate or "outside" effort marginalizes its potential impact. CEOs need to grapple with the degree of inclusion and communication the foundation board could be privy to from the healthcare organization and the degree of collaboration that could exist with the governing board. CEOs who are willing and able to treat the foundation board as one of equal stature but separate function from the governing board can create a new level of board ownership and engagement.

Individual board leaders and the governing and foundation boards as collective bodies can provide a clear competitive advantage in advancing philanthropy. Without the support of these leaders, fund development efforts hit a performance ceiling that cannot be broken by the brightest and most committed foundation staff. Therefore, the engagement of these leaders by the CEO significantly leverages her involvement, as her influence becomes the stone thrown in the water that creates ongoing ripples all around it.

Facilitate Physician Engagement

Development executives know grateful patients are a core constituency to foster as prospective donors, and research validates that physicians hold the greatest influence in connecting grateful patients to the healthcare mission. While some compel involvement in development from employed physicians, many physicians remain independent contractors with the choice to participate in fund development activities or not. However, whether physicians are employed or autonomous, the CEO has outsize influence in inspiring leadership and creating ownership to enable their informed, invested, and impactful involvement.

The CEO is confronted with multiple reasons to strengthen hospital-physician partnerships. The Affordable Care Act (ACA) is spurring greater integration with physicians with the realization that more effective care delivery will require a team approach. Many hospitals are launching deep collaborations with physicians to pursue the "Triple Aim" to improve quality, safety, and satisfaction; to improve the health of populations; and to reduce the per capita cost of healthcare. There is also a new understanding that hospital–physician collaboration will be required to successfully shift from a model of intermittent care to a model of ongoing relationships to help people stay well. As the CEO pursues physician partnership across these top-level priorities, philanthropy can be placed in context as a force for powering not only these shared goals but also for driving innovation in programs, technology, and patient care environment.

The CEO recognizes physicians live in an evidence-based world where data is a key language. Physicians are trained to focus on outcomes, protocols, benchmarks, and other numbers and processes that substantiate the need for certain actions or approaches. CEOs talk this language as well and can effectively answer the question of *why* physician involvement is an appropriate and value-added effort that merits their attention.

The CEO values being a primary point of engagement to physicians, since the quality of a CEO's relationships with physicians has become a hallmark of the effective leader. In seeking the involvement of physicians, the CEO has the most traction in recruiting specific physicians to specific endeavors, such as personally asking a respected physician leader to be a champion for a funding priority in his area of practice. CEOs can also affirm the value of physician participation by honoring physicians who participate in public and hospital forums that matter to them, such as medical staff or section meetings that include their professional peers and in the boardroom that represents the wider community. By linking the CEO into physician engagement, it aligns with the CEO's existing priorities to drive better hospital–physician partnerships while simultaneously deploying the hospital's best messengers to a high-value task.

Overcome Obstacles to Participation

Despite the considerable influence of the CEO, many CEOs express reluctance to get involved in fund development activities. CEOs often attribute their hesitation to:

- lack of knowledge of the financial potential of philanthropy,
- lack of comfort in how to be effective in a fund development role, or
- lack of available time to participate.

Overcoming a lack of knowledge about the financial potential of philanthropy is the easiest because it is a simple information issue. Basics the CEO must know include:

- The Association for Healthcare Philanthropy (AHP) says healthcare organizations in the United States raise almost $9 billion annually.[41]
- AHP says it costs $0.31 at the median to raise $1.00 from giving.[5]
- Benchmarking services, like the AHP Performance Benchmarking Service, allow organizations to compare their financial performance and potential against cohorts based on a variety of variables.
- The ROI achievable from philanthropy typically far outstrips the ROI possible from any clinical service line.
- Healthcare organizations performing at the median operating margin at the writing of this chapter would have to generate $21.88 million from operations to put $1.0 million on the bottom line, while healthcare fund development organizations performing at the median would need to raise $1.44 million to get $1.0 million to the bottom line.[42]
- There is no diminishing point of return for investing in fund development: the more an organization invests, the more it generates.

---

41 Association for Healthcare Philanthropy, AHP Report on Giving FY12, October 2013
42 HealthLeaders Fact File Hospital Financial Trends July/August 2013

11 Reasons CEOs Don't Help:

- I don't want the healthcare organization to appear weak.
- I don't see the potential in philanthropy.
- My plate is more than full; I don't have the time.
- I hired the foundation staff to do that stuff.
- The board has other priorities for my time.
- I don't feel like I have the skills to be successful.
- I would be embarrassed to ask.
- I'm not comfortable with the social interaction involved.
- I don't understand the rules around HIPAA.
- I don't socialize with wealthy people.
- I'm not sure how to help.

The CEO and Solicitation

Most CEOs are high-performing individuals, so lack of comfort can be a significant barrier to participation. Some CEOs avoid solicitation because they don't feel they have the tools, training, or interpersonal skills. It's helpful to remind the CEO that on a solicitation call, she would most often be the voice of the vision of the organization to explain the solution that is proposed, the due diligence behind the planning process, the reason the healthcare organization feels it is best prepared to advance the solution, and the anticipated community benefit of the initiative moving forward. The CEO would also share plans and timelines for implementation and disclose the healthcare organization's own financial commitment for the implementation and sustainability of the project. CEOs don't need to avoid solicitation calls out of fear they will be under the pressure to close transactions.

Overcoming a lack of comfort can be a training issue or a matter of engaging the CEO in right-fit roles that align with his natural talents and skills. There are a variety of resources for training executives about philanthropy that allow leaders to put philanthropy and their individual role within it in context.

However, *Harvard Business Review* points out that it is unfair to expect the CEO to be a master at everything: "Top executives, the thinking goes, should have the intellectual capacity to make sense of unfathomably complex issues, the imaginative powers to paint a vision of the future that generates everyone's enthusiasm, the operational know-how to translate strategy into concrete plans, and the interpersonal skills to foster commitment to undertakings that could cost people's jobs should they fail. Unfortunately, no single person can possibly live up to those standards. It's time to end the myth of the complete leader: the flawless person at the top who's got it all figured out."[43]

With this in mind, activities for the CEO need to be tailored to his strengths and abilities as well as his constraints. This means there is great merit to having an honest conversation with the CEO about the variety of high-value external roles that make up the spectrum of the development process as well as the high-impact internal roles that support and facilitate the work. Then discuss the activities the CEO really must be part of, those that could be fulfilled by other surrogates, and those that play to the CEO's strengths. Then you can have an agreed-upon plan for how key work will get done.

Ironically, there's a good chance the final argument—not having time—is closely related to the other two reasons—lack of knowledge and lack of skills. There is no doubt today's executives are incredibly busy with the many obligations of running a complex organization. However, there are certain types of things that tend to fall off people's calendars more easily. People don't spend time on things they don't perceive to be important. People also avoid activities they aren't confident

---

43 "In Praise of the Incomplete Leader", Debora Ancona, Thomas W. Malone, Wanda J. Orlikowski, Peter M. Senge, Harvard Business Review, February 2007, http://hbr.org/2007/02/in-praise-of-the-incomplete-leader, accessed April 6, 2014

they have the training or skills to do, since they don't want to expose their limitations. When reasons like this start piling up, it's easy to see how fund development activities fall into the deep, dark, calendar abyss. However, not allocating time comes at a big opportunity cost and may create a self-fulfilling prophecy when a lack of leadership engagement becomes a lack of performance.

Share a Common Language

To engage the CEO, development leaders must talk in a language executives hear and understand: the language of business. Too many CEOs say they see healthcare philanthropy as a *soft* or *social* endeavor. They say development staff reminds them this is "an art and not a science." However, that's just not the case. While relationships will always be at the core of philanthropy, the practice and profession of fund development has the benefit of best practices, benchmarks, metrics, data analysis, and processes to fuel diligence. These resources allow development professionals to validate the efficiency and effectiveness of their programs and to forecast their financial impact on the healthcare organization. By demonstrating that fund development is a management function with clear and strategic bottom-line implications, the perception of development work can be elevated from a frivolous endeavor characterized by galas and golf tournaments to a strategic revenue opportunity that merits being on the leadership agenda.

Using the language of business does not cut the heart out of this work or dishonor valued relationships with donors. Work as a fund development professional is always rooted in purpose and in the nobility of this calling. However, advancing the practice of fund development with diligence is a manifestation of good stewardship. Business consultant and author Jim Collins expresses this idea well in his monograph, "Good to Great and the Social Sectors," when he says, "A culture of discipline is not a principle of *business*; it is a principle of *greatness*."[44]

---

44 Jim Collins, Good to Great and the Social Sectors, Excerpt http://www.jimcollins.com/books/g2g-ss.html

It is time to pursue greatness, and greatness is within grasp when healthcare fund development organizations can engage CEOs to build a strategic, cultural, and tactical platform for performance and to galvanize the commitment and action of key advocates to elevate this noble work.

Executive Summary

- CEO engagement in both practical and symbolic roles is critical to optimize fund development efforts.
- While many internal roles in advancing philanthropy can be moved forward in a lesser capacity by others, the influence and expectation-setting of the CEO is unmatchable in building the internal platform for performance.
- The CEO's most leveraged role is in engaging and empowering board and physician advocates, and emphasis should be placed on conveying the strategic importance of philanthropy and on making specific calls to action.
- Development leaders must talk in a language executives hear and understand—the language of business—to demonstrate that fund development is a management function with best practices, benchmarks, metrics, data analysis, and processes to fuel diligence rather than a decorative, social function.

Discussion

1. What impact could CEO engagement have on your fund development program in terms of engaging key advocates, positioning development within the healthcare organization, achieving alignment between organizational strategy and funding priorities, accessing information, receiving adequate financial investment, etc.?

2. What keeps your CEO from actively advancing philanthropy now? Lack of understanding of the potential? Not a priority relative to other tasks? Concern that fundraising makes the healthcare organization look weak? Personal embarrassment to ask?

3. How do you engage with your CEO now around the role and impact of the CEO in philanthropy? Do you have opportunities to elevate your dialogue by talking about philanthropy using the language of business?

4. How could you enhance the chief executive officer–chief development officer partnership? Do you have the base of trust, mutual respect, and consistent communication you need? If not, how can you develop it?

5. How could the CEO assist in creating an organizational culture that supports philanthropy and gets people engaged from the front line to the boardroom to the exam room in promoting the healthcare mission as a valuable endeavor, worthy of charitable investment?

6. Are expectations for participation in philanthropy formally included in the CEO's job description or part of the tasks for which the CEO is annually evaluated? If not, if philanthropy were formally recognized as an organizational priority, would it be easier for the CEO to allocate time to his active involvement?

Author Bio

Betsy Chapin Taylor, FAHP, leads the healthcare philanthropy consulting firm Accordant Philanthropy, which fosters the leveraged engagement of executives, board members, and physicians in advancing philanthropy. She also serves as a faculty member of the American College of Healthcare Executives, teaching CEOs how to advance philanthropy as a key revenue resource. She is author of the book *Healthcare Philanthropy: Advance Charitable Giving to Your*

Organization's Mission, which explores healthcare philanthropy from a CEO's perspective, published by Health Administration Press and the Association for Healthcare Philanthropy. She is also the author of the study guide "Advancing the CEO's Role in Healthcare Philanthropy," published by the American College of Healthcare Executives.

Leveraging the Influence of Board Members

Betsy Chapin Taylor, FAHP

MANY HEALTHCARE ORGANIZATIONS fail to fully engage foundation and governing board members to advance philanthropy. Some perceive fund development as a low-value, social endeavor that doesn't merit significant leadership involvement. Many downplay the importance of the role out of concern that raising money is off-putting to board members. Others strip philanthropy from the governing board agenda and relegate it exclusively to the foundation board. Many allow a painful disconnect to exist between the roles board members are asked to fulfill and the roles these leaders have the passion, comfort, or skills to do well. To realize the abundant potential philanthropy offers, it's time to focus on meaningful board engagement across both the foundation board and governing board. To do so, organizations must embrace philanthropy as a noble endeavor, recognize philanthropy as a governance responsibility, leverage the power of social capital, tap into individual purpose, and provide meaningful opportunities for involvement.

Philanthropy is Noble

Deep board member engagement in fund development begins by abandoning the transactional, fundraising paradigm of yesterday and positioning philanthropy as a purpose-filled, values-driven, and noble endeavor. In advancing philanthropy, there is no tin cup to rattle, no arm to twist, and nobody to coerce. Instead, board members have the privilege to foster relationships with like-minded people to fulfill a shared purpose. Arthur C. Brooks frames the value of this role in *The New York Times*; he says, "Donors possess two disconnected commodities: material wealth and sincere convictions. Alone, these commodities are difficult to combine. But fundraisers facilitate an alchemy of virtue: They empower those with financial resources to convert the dross of their money into the gold of a better society."[45]

Part of Our Rich and Vibrant Roots

Statesman Benjamin Franklin first positioned health-care philanthropy as a civic responsibility to be championed by community leadership volunteers. Franklin established a hospital board in 1752 to raise charitable funds to create our nation's first hospital. Trustees were chosen based upon personal wealth and civic connections to foster charitable support. Franklin's philosophy was that each man should be asked to give in a way commensurate to his own means and to present the vision to others with a request for a specific amount based upon the donor's means. [46]

45 Brooks, Arthur C., "Why Fundraising Is Fun", The New York Times, March 29, 2014
46 Brenmer, Robert H., American Philanthropy, University of Chicago Press, 1988

Philanthropy is a Governance Role

Most discussions about boards and fund development focus exclusively on the roles and responsibilities of the foundation board. This is because most healthcare governing boards have viewed fund development as an ancillary activity, and many have fully delegated their development roles to the foundation board. This is understandable from a historical perspective since fundraising was often perceived as a softer, social endeavor, and donor contributions were often used to fund value-added rather than strategically-important initiatives. However, seizing the opportunity philanthropy presents means organizations must engage both foundation and governing boards to secure the breadth and depth of leadership commitment needed.

Philanthropy has strategic and fiduciary implications that necessitate its inclusion on the governing board agenda. Healthcare governing boards balance the need to meet expanding community healthcare needs with the reality of constricting financial resources. Strategic and fiduciary responsibilities dovetail as the board sets and executes upon strategy that requires adequate financial resources to power the plans. These complementary fiduciary roles have been increasingly difficult to reconcile as slim bottom lines reduce dollars to invest in the organization's advancement, and the implementation of health reform brings additional financial risk as the way hospitals provide care and get paid for doing so fundamentally changes. In this new financial landscape, healthcare organizations must develop revenue streams that can ensure their vibrant future. With philanthropy delivering a strong return on investment and a reliable revenue stream, it merits the status of an essential revenue resource worthy of board attention and support.

Beyond the board's financial and strategic roles, there is a third mode of effective governance that shifts the board from an "ubermanager" to a force to add significant value. This critical third element is a "generative" mindset that seeks to create better approaches to further the mission, to drive innovation, and to capture value.[47] This generative mindset

---

47 Chait, Richard; Ryan, William; Taylor, Babara, "Governance as Leadership: Reframing the Work of Nonprofit Boards", 2004

Governing Board Roles:

- Cement an organizational commitment to advance philanthropy
- Recognize advancing philanthropy as a valued role of the CEO
- Position development as a strategic revenue resource
- Foster an organizational culture to advance philanthropy
- Ensure alignment between funding priorities and organizational strategy
- Define a unique, valuable, and specific role for charitable giving
- Allocate adequate budget resources to fuel both capacity and growth
- Provide input toward a compelling case for support
- Track performance measures for philanthropy
- Recognize the charitable underpinning of the organization in its brand
- Leverage connections, open doors, and secure donor commitments
- Give at a level commensurate with your ability and interest

Foundation Board Roles:

- Participate in the full spectrum of donor engagement activities
- Select strategically aligned and donor-appropriate funding priorities
- Evaluate, shape, and approve the case for support
- Approve fund development campaigns and goals
- Monitor progress toward development goals and objectives
- Drive accountability and refinement by utilizing benchmarking
- Identify and engage other leadership volunteers as advocates
- Provide oversight for management and use of charitable funds
- Approve allocations to the healthcare organization
- Support the leadership of the CDO in her management role
- Give at a level commensurate with your ability and interest

elevates the focus from holding the organization accountable to driving consequential work. It is within this generative space that boards could find great resonance in advancing philanthropy as an opportunity to embrace the charitable underpinnings of the healthcare mission, to bring core values to life, to invite the community to take ownership, and to secure dollars to drive new opportunities and greater impact.

Philanthropy is a governance role in which boards are uniquely positioned to add value. The book *Governance as Leadership* makes a distinction between work that requires *no* board, *any* board, or *this* board.[48] Work that requires *no* board is often management work that has been sent to the board inappropriately or for rubber-stamping. Work that requires *any* board could be managed by any group of responsible individuals; for example, the board of another complex nonprofit could likely review the organization's financial reports or policies effectively. Then there is work that requires *this* board: it not only takes diligent and well-intentioned people but also requires those with care for the mission, sensitivity to the critical issues that impact its future, and ownership of the outcomes. Under this standard, philanthropy is a high-impact board role because of the knowledge and passion needed to do it well.

Social Capital as a Strategic Asset

It's no secret board members are uniquely positioned to enhance philanthropy. While boards almost always work as a collective body, some of the most impactful roles in philanthropy are tied to individual engagement and performance. Board members are ideally suited to initiate or cement significant relationships and to secure outsize gifts. Board members carry influence that isn't duplicated anywhere else in the organization. Board members have unmatched credibility as advocates, since it is clear their only vested interest in the organization is in the community benefit it provides. Board members also tend to be true

---

48   Chait, Richard; Ryan, William; Taylor, Babara, "Governance as Leadership: Reframing the Work of Nonprofit Boards", 2004. p 170

The Credibility to Ask

Clearly for a board member to be effective in this outreach and advocacy role, she must have made a personal financial commitment at a level appropriate to her ability and interest to validate her credibility as an asker.

peers of potential donors who can inspire and challenge others through their own personal charitable gifts.

Widespread anecdotal evidence lauds the influence of board members in advancing key relationships for philanthropy, but there is also quantitative information that validates this elevated effectiveness. A study at Virginia Mason Medical Center in Seattle, Washington, found donor prospects involved in the organization by board members gave gifts that were almost five times larger than those given by staff-connected prospects and after fewer interactions.[49] A study by The Advisory Board Company found "volunteers have a much easier time than staff getting in the door" and points out volunteers successfully secure appointments on about nine out of 10 attempts, while staff secure a meeting about two times for every 10 attempts.[50] Performance differences like this have considerable implications for the number of individuals an organization could involve and secure commitments from in a board-driven model.

Board members achieve heightened performance because of the *social capital* associated with their diverse network of social, civic, and business connections. Harvard University professor and political scientist Robert Putnam explains, "Whereas *physical capital* refers to physical objects and *human capital* refers to the properties of individuals, *social capital* refers to connections among individuals—social networks and the norms of reciprocity and trustworthiness that arise from them."[51]

49 Jachim, Jeanne, "Major Gift Officers: A Valuable Commodity—are We Using and Evaluating Them Well?", AHP Journal, Fall 2010

50 The Advisory Board Company, "Re-envisioning the Alliance", p.2, 2009

51 Putnam, Robert Putnam, Bowling Alone: The collapse and revival of American community, New York: Simon and Schuster, p19, 2000

Putnam says each person's network is the embodiment of past success at collaboration, and these positive experiences working together provide the confidence to collaborate again. So social capital, like all other forms of capital, has real and significant value.

Social capital serves a variety of important functions between trusted individuals. Most significantly, social capital can act as "social superglue" to foster collaboration or as "social WD-40" to facilitate interactions going smoothly.[52] Social capital leverages the interconnectedness of people, acquired trust, shared values, social norms, and moral obligations to allow people to effectively come together to advance shared objectives; and social capital is an essential commodity to amplify the voice of and secure access for the organization.

The concept of social capital is consistent with other findings about the most impactful roles of board members in fund development. A study from the Nonprofit Research Collaborative found "board members serve two primary functions: helping the organization reach new prospective donors (access) and indicating the organization's value to the community by their own association with the group (signaling)."[53] These access and signaling roles rely on social capital to extend trust in the board member's reputation to become trust in the healthcare organization.

Having an authentic way to establish trust is especially important in a world where both trust and genuine relationships are a rare commodity. People today are overwhelmed with automated personalization and customized communication, and *Stanford Social Innovation Review* points out "people are growing increasingly intolerant of messages from people they don't really know... They are increasingly limiting their attention to messages from trusted friends and business colleagues."[54] Having a board member cut through this noise to legitimize the nonprofit is irreplaceable.

---

52 Putnam, Robert Putnam, Bowling Alone: The collapse and revival of American community, New York: Simon and Schuster, pp 22-23, 2000

53 Nonprofit Research Collaborative, "Special Report: Engaging Board Members in Fundraising", p4, September 2012

54 Simpson, David, "Peer to Peer Fundraising Deserves Top-Level Focus and Resources", Stanford Social Innovation Review, May 12, 2011

Board engagement to foster relationships also helps overcome the idiosyncrasies of human nature. For example, the field of behavioral economics shows people do not behave *rationally* but behave *irrationally in predictable ways*. This leads donors to make emotional, intuitive giving decisions that they then validate logically to justify the decision. This same phenomenon extends to the power and influence of the solicitor. *Harvard Business Review* explains that "weak market forces exist" in the nonprofit sector that mean donor choice is "often influenced by personal relationships… rather than by organizational performance."[55] So demonstrated impact doesn't mean much if you don't have the connectivity of the right person to carry the message.

Ultimately, the sum of each board member's social capital and personal network creates a powerful force for connectivity with donors and an organic, vibrant, and ever-expanding circle of friends for the organization.

Purpose Trumps Obligation

When board members utilize their social capital to advance the organization, they use their own reputation as collateral to vouch for the organization. This is a commitment few would make out of simple obligation. It is an undertaking that won't be fulfilled simply because it was on a punchlist of things a board member should do. Instead, extending one's reputation must be consistent with a board member's values and individual purpose.

Most board members serve to achieve a positive impact, to advance their core values, and to pursue their passion—and achieving full engagement requires tapping into this individual purpose. Building engagement on a platform that respects individual purpose creates a new board engagement paradigm that shifts the focus from a litany of tasks to check off to deeper motivations to fulfill.

Bestselling business author Dan Pink's book *Drive* says the secret

---

55 Bradach, Jeffrey L, et al, "Delivering on the Promise of Nonprofits", Harvard Business Review, December 2008

Recruit for Purpose

A board engagement paradigm rooted in purpose presents a recruitment issue. If board members join at the direction of their employer, to pad their resume, to seek business leads, or out of any other form of self-interest, connecting to purpose will not motivate them. The aim to serve must be outward-focused and consistent with each member's core values, passion, and purpose. That's because "passion for mission" is a basic quality on the level of someone having blood running through his veins.

to achieving a high level of individual performance is in meeting the individual's deeply human needs. The book explores four decades of scientific work on human motivation to illuminate three specific elements that motivate people. He says each person's own intrinsic inner drive pushes him to seek *autonomy* to direct his own life and control his own decisions, *mastery* to learn and create new things, and *purpose* to do better by himself and his world. He says true motivation to action depends on first meeting these three very basic, human needs.[56]

Gallup research further validates a universal desire for our individual lives to have a purpose and to matter. When asked, "How important to you is the belief that your life is meaningful or has purpose," an astounding 98% say it is important to them. They want their lives to make a difference. They want meaning. They want purpose.[57]

There is a difference between collective purpose and individual purpose. The board has a *collective* purpose to support the mission of the nonprofit healthcare organization. However, the aim here is to connect to each board member's *individual* purpose that reflects her own values and her vision of the impact she wants to make on the world. Organizations uncover the purpose of each individual board member through asking key questions, such as:

56 Pink, Daniel H, Drive: The Surprising Truth About What Motivates Us, Penguin, 2011
57 Wagner, Rodd and Harter, Jim, Gallup Business Journal, "The Eighth Element of Great Managing", December 13, 2007

- What first kindled your interest in our mission?
- What personal experiences have you had with the organization?
- What do you believe in and care about that connects you to the mission here?
- What are your core values that could be extended through this work?
- What impact do you want to have on this work and on this world?
- What about our mission gives you hope or joy?
- What legacy do you want to leave here?

Having one-on-one, meaningful conversations with leaders moves you from having a group of undifferentiated members to discovering the magic found in each unique and passionate individual. It allows you to find out what motivates each person, moves her or makes her want to get engaged. It provides an audacious opportunity to fundamentally change the way you partner with your boards.

Enable Advocate Success

Few leaders agree to serve on a board because they want the opportunity to ask others for money, and you know many of your board advocates do not feel comfortable in the role of asking. In fact, 59% of board members express being uncomfortable asking others to give, and they share two primary concerns:[58]

- Damage to their relationships by asking for a gift and
- Failure in the task because they don't "know how" to successfully engage others.

This first concern often stems from a perception that asking for money will involve coercion, *quid pro quo*, or pressure tactics. The second concern is common because board members tend to be high-performing

---

58 BoardSource, 2012 BoardSource Nonprofit Governance Index, p. 17, 2012, http://www.thenonprofitpartnership.org/files/board-source-governance-2012.pdf

Be Honest about Expectations

Expectations of board members for participation in philanthropy can be a sensitive subject. Yet, the effective deployment of board members relies on setting clear and specific expectations at the outset. Board members feel misled or poorly utilized when the organization fails to be forthright about fund development duties at recruitment. While many organizations downplay the development role in order to secure agreement to join the board, this can perpetuate the idea that development is not important and allow the entire board to largely abandon the development role.

people who don't want to be "set up for failure" by not having the resources to be successful. However, given the importance of engaging board members to build relationships, this gap must be bridged.

Development executives, along with board leaders, must proactively enable the success and confident participation of members by providing actionable information and tools to demystify development, to place the role in context, and to address specific situations. Board members also need to be empowered with the understanding that their relationship-building work does not need to be done with expertise but with authenticity: A board member's peers do not value having someone who is an expert in asking; they seek a genuine conversation with a person they trust. In advocating for the organization, there is a very simple formula from the sales world that is relatable to a board member's development role. The gist is that a board member's role is never to convince anyone to give but is to present an opportunity and listen to understand the donor's intentions and needs. *Forbes* magazine expresses the idea simply as "SEA":

- Sincerity: Listen without an agenda;
- Ethics: Don't aim to talk someone into anything but to uncover intent; and

- Asking: Serve others by asking questions to aid their decisions.[59]

Board members deserve to participate in value-added activities that are also aligned with their own strengths, talents, comfort zone, interests, and constraints. Simply, there doesn't need to be a one-size-fits-all, lockstep approach to board roles in fund development. High-value activities for board members might include:

- Identifying those with likely interest and financial ability to participate,
- Qualifying interest to ensure someone is genuinely a good prospect,
- Sharing stories of individuals whose lives were touched or changed,
- Illuminating that the organization is a nonprofit that exists to provide community benefit,
- Making introductions or otherwise opening doors to those in their network,
- Educating prospective donors about the organization's vision and initiatives,
- Engaging current and prospective donors in the life of the organization,
- Asking donors to make a financial commitment to support the mission, or
- Stewarding donors to demonstrate thanks and fidelity in fulfilling their intent.

Given the broad spectrum of meaningful development activities, board members should be able to choose amongst various roles to create their own engagement plan—rather than having everyone fulfill a set list of responsibilities such as: 1) identify 10 prospects, 2) make five face-to-face visits, and 3) fill one table at the gala.

---

59   Michael, Sharon, "3 Powerful Skills You Must Have to Succeed in Sales", August 22, 2011, Forbes, http://www.forbes.com/sites/womensmedia/2011/08/22/3-powerful-skills-you-must-have-to-succeed-in-sales)

A famous experiment showed the value of giving people choice. In the experiment, half of the group was given a preprinted lottery ticket, while the other half of the group was given a blank piece of paper and a pen to write down lottery numbers they chose themselves. Before the alleged drawing was to occur, researchers offered to buy back the tickets. What they found was that those who had preprinted tickets with numbers assigned to them would readily part with the tickets. However, those who chose numbers for themselves were more reluctant to sell, and wanted five times more in exchange for the tickets. The takeaway here is clear and simple: we are all more committed to a plan we craft for ourselves.[60] Allowing choice enables greater ownership of the work to be done and allows board members to select activities with which they are both comfortable and committed.

Board Engagement Takes Your Commitment

Connecting to purpose and providing right-fit opportunities to get active provides a path to deep engagement for board members, but it requires deliberate and proactive allocations of time and attention by development leaders. This can be a challenge for the busy executive. However, a study by CompassPoint Nonprofit Services and the Meyer Foundation shows the more effort nonprofit leaders put into supporting their boards, the happier they are with the board's performance—yet, more than half of nonprofit leaders say they spend 10 hours or fewer per month supporting their boards.[61] Ten hours may sound significant, but that is just 30 minutes per workday. In *The Chronicle of Philanthropy*, study author Rick Moyers notes, "Some executive directors view their work with the board as an unwelcome distraction from their 'real' work. For that reason, they spend as little time on the board as possible, at the same time wondering out loud why the board can't be more self-sufficient and why it doesn't give them more help. However, this 'neglect and grumble' strategy doesn't

---

60 Keller, Scott, HBR.org, "Increase Your Team's Motivation Five-Fold", April 26, 2012
61 Moyers, Rick, Daring to Lead 2011 Brief 3: The Board Paradox, San Francisco, CA; Compass Point Nonprofit Services and the Meyer Foundation, 2011

improve board performance. To get more out of their boards, executives need to invest more time."[62]

Logically, you know investing time to orient and support a board member unleashes her potential. However, many organizations still opt to try to do all the work themselves. This not only removes a key lever to performance from the organization but also denies board members an opportunity to be part of impactful work for the organization. It also sets up a chain of frustration, with development executives bemoaning that the board doesn't help and board members saying that the organization doesn't ask them to do anything substantive. Building an engaged and inspired board takes effort. However, the multiplier effect of doing so outweighs the effort required.

A Call to Purpose-Driven Action

It is time to prioritize board engagement to achieve a new level of impact for your organization. This requires recognizing philanthropy as a governance role that merits being on the agenda of both the governing and foundation boards. It entails leveraging each board member's valuable, personal networks to gain access, build trust, and amplify the message of the organization. It requires tapping into each member's personal purpose to harness real motivation. Finally, it requires commitment to align opportunities with board members' natural strengths, to give them the ability to choose how they will participate, and to provide them with resources and support. By changing your board engagement paradigm, organizations can experience deeper connections with donors and more meaningful partnerships with some of the organization's greatest advocates.

---

62 Moyers, Rick, "Executive Directors Should Invest More Time on Their Boards", Chronicle of Philanthropy, August 23, 2011.

Executive Summary

- Philanthropy has strategic and fiduciary implications that necessitate the attention and involvement of the governing board in addition to the foundation board.
- Board members are uniquely positioned to successfully foster the engagement of community donors because of the *social capital* associated with their diverse network of social, civic, and business connections.
- Board members deserve the opportunity to select to participate in development activities aligned with their own passion, purpose, strengths, talents, comfort zone, and constraints.
- Development executives must dedicate the time and attention to proactively enable the confident participation of board members by providing actionable information and tools to demystify development, to place the role in context, and to support success.

Discussion

Questions for Fund Development Executives

1. What do you know about each foundation board member and governing board member as an individual rather than as a member of a group? How can you better understand their unique motivations, passions, and purposes?
2. How can you engage board members in choosing specific opportunities to advance healthcare philanthropy that are consistent with their individual talents, interests, passions, purposes, and constraints?
3. How will you support, encourage, and affirm board members in fulfilling their role? What resources,

training, and staff support make a commensurate investment in the impact you seek?

4. How can you collaborate with board leadership to develop a clear list of specific expectations for participation in philanthropy that the board requires of its own members and that has an accompanying mechanism for driving accountability?

5. Is your healthcare organization's governing board keenly aware of the financial rationale for philanthropy and the role giving can play in advancing the healthcare organization? If not, how can you proactively inform their understanding of the opportunity?

Questions for the Governing Board or Foundation Board

1. How does fund development fit into your concept of good governance?

2. How can you better align the healthcare organization and foundation?

3. How can you improve the impact of philanthropy in the organization?

4. How will you become more intentional about fund development efforts?

5. How can the governing board and foundation board better collaborate?

6. What expectations do you have for board participation in philanthropy?

7. What training, skills, and resources does the board need to be successful?

Questions for Individual Board Members

1. How does advancing the healthcare organization align with your core values?

2. Do you believe in the organization enough to introduce your friends to it?

3. How could you effectively use your social capital to advance the mission?

4. How can you silence your squeamishness about solicitation?

5. How will you sharpen your skills to increase your comfort and effectiveness?

6. What development activities fit your purpose, talents, and constraints?

Author Bio

Betsy Chapin Taylor, FAHP, leads the healthcare philanthropy consulting firm Accordant Philanthropy, which fosters the leveraged engagement of executives, board members, and physicians in advancing philanthropy. She is author of the monograph "Boards and Philanthropy: Developing the Next-Curve Revenue Source for Health Care" from the American Hospital Association's Center for Healthcare Governance. She is also author of the book *Healthcare Philanthropy: Advance Charitable Giving to Your Organization's Mission*, published by Health Administration Press and the Association for Healthcare Philanthropy.

Engage Physicians and Create a Culture of Gratitude
Chad Gobel and Alisa Stetzer

ONE OF THE GREATEST opportunities for revenue growth in a hospital or health system is through philanthropic investments from patients who are grateful for the care and compassion they have received. In most cases, the untapped philanthropic potential of grateful patients for a hospital or health system is in the millions of dollars *annually*.

To achieve this growth, hospital leaders, especially physicians, need to think and act differently toward philanthropy. Today, most hospital leaders and physicians consider philanthropy a financial transaction. It's not surprising, since that is how philanthropy leaders talk about their work. Development organizations measure success by how much money has been raised. You talk about the size of gifts you've closed. You measure return on investment and cost to raise a dollar. Yet with grateful patients, it's not about a transaction; it's about a transformational experience.

Part of the Healing Process

Grateful patient philanthropy programs, as their name suggests, are a way for patients to express their gratitude through philanthropy to the physicians, nurses, and other caregivers. The donor's gratitude is in direct response to the high quality, clinical excellence, and exceptional experience they have had in the course of their healthcare encounter.[63] These grateful patients have had the kind of care from providers every hospital and health system is working hard to achieve.

Grateful patients will often say to care providers, "What may seem ordinary to you is extraordinary to me. I feel so fortunate to have had such exceptional care." This patient gratitude and its resulting philanthropy are tangible outcomes of the myriad ways organizations are working to drive exceptional patient experience.

Gratitude is Good for Health

Clinical research provides compelling evidence to promote the role of philanthropy in patient encounters. Engaging in expressions of gratitude, such as those expressed by a grateful patient, has been linked to an increased ability to cope with stress; a stronger immune function; quicker recovery from illness; lower blood pressure; increased feelings of connectedness, which improve relationships and well-being, greater joy; optimism; and increased generosity and compassion.[64] In a review article published by Harvard Health Publications in November 2011, they put it quite succinctly: "expressing thanks may be one of the simplest ways to feel better."[65]

Happy Patients and Improved Health

When those expressions of gratitude are linked with a wish to make a

63 Stewart, Rosalyn, Wolfe, Leah, Flynn, John, Carrese, Joseph, and Wright, Scott. 2011. "Success in Grateful Patient Philanthropy: Insights from Experienced Physicians." American Journal of Medicine. 12: 1181-1185.

64 Emmons, Robert. 2010. "Why is Gratitude Good?" Greater Good: The Science of Meaningful Life. Online article. November 16, 2010. Accessed February 28, 2014 online at http://greatergood.berkeley.edu/article/item/why_gratitude_is_good /

65 "In Praise of Gratitude". 2011. The Harvard Mental Health Letter, November 2011. http://www.health.harvard.edu/newsletters/Harvard_Mental_Health_Letter/2011/November/in-praise-of-gratitude.

philanthropic gift, it causes happiness. A study published in *Science* by Harvard Business School in 2008 showed spending money on others causes happiness more than spending on oneself.[66] People who participate in charitable giving are 43% more likely to report they are "very happy" than non-givers, while non-givers are three and a half times more likely than givers to report they are "not happy at all."[67] People who give and experience happiness are more likely to give again in the future, causing more happiness and making them more likely to give again, in a self-perpetuating cycle.[68]

Happiness has also been linked to good health. Beyond the immediate elevated mood experienced when people feel happy, happiness has been shown to add as much as nine years to one's life expectancy[69] and can reduce blood pressure and the risk of cardiovascular disease.[70] Similarly, charitable giving has been linked to many physical health improvements, including a stronger immune response, decreased levels of stress hormones, a quicker cardiovascular recovery from stress, increased long-term survival in HIV/AIDS patients, decreased blood pressure, and decreased viral loads.[71] The suggestion has also been made that charitable giving at high rates of frequency may protect patients from the onset of new health issues when faced with a new stressor (Poulin, *et al.* 2013). Finally, charitable giving was shown to reduce overall mortality rate in older adults by as much as 47%.[72]

66   Dunn, Elizabeth, Aknin, Lara and Norton, Michael. 2008. "Spending Money on Others Promotes Happiness." Science. 319: 1687-1688.

67   Brooks, Arthur. 2007. Who Really Cares: The Surprising Truth about Compassionate Conservatism. New York: Basic Books.

68   Aknin, Lara, Dunn, Elizabeth and Norton, Michael. 2012. "Happiness Runs in Circular Motion: Evidence for a Positive Feedback Loop Between Prosocial Spending and Happiness." Journal of Happiness Studies. 13: 347-355.

69   Emmons, Robert. 2007. Thanks! How the New Science of Gratitude Can Make you Happier. Boston: Houghton Mifflin.

70   Fredrickson, Barbara. 1998. "What Good are Positive Emotions?" Review of General Psychology. 2(3): 300-316.

71   Konrath, Sara. 2013. "The Power of Philanthropy and Volunteering". In Wellbeing: A Complete Reference Guide. Volume 6: Interventions and Policies to Enhance Wellbeing. Felicia Huppert and Cary Cooper (Eds). Malden, MA: Wiley Press.

72   Okun, Morris, WanHeung Yeung, Ellen and Brown, Stephanie. 2013. "Volunteering by

Reduced Suffering

People who suffer significant losses in the course of their care are particularly motivated to help others not *despite* their difficult experiences, but specifically *because* of them. In order to survive a traumatic event, a key task in effective healing is to restore "shattered assumptions" of the world and to find new meaning and value in life.[73] Giving is a way grateful patients find that meaning, purpose, value, and connection.[74] Author and Holocaust survivor Viktor Frankl suggested, "In some ways, suffering ceases to be suffering at the moment it finds a meaning."[75]

Charitable acts have been shown to decrease depression and post-traumatic stress in bereaved spouses and patients with chronic illnesses one year later.[76] In turn, positive emotions generated by the philanthropic act of giving, like all acts of gratitude, help people better manage stress and make better self-care decisions (e.g., exercise more and for longer periods of time[77]) which drives improved physical health. For patients and families who have suffered great losses, there may be an even greater need and rationale to engage in philanthropic giving.

The Cost of Not Giving

When clinicians and care providers respond to a grateful patient by saying, "You don't need to give; we're just glad you're better," the

---

Older Adults and Risk of Mortality: A Meta-Analysis". Psychology and Aging. 28(2): 564–577.

73   , Johanna. 2009. "Altruism Born of Suffering and Prosocial Behavior Following Adverse Life Events: A Review and Conceptualization." Social Justice Research. 22: 53-97.

74   Janoff-Bulman, Ronnie. 1992. Shattered Assumptions: Towards A New Psychology of Trauma. New York: Free Press.

75   Frankl, Viktor. 1958. Man's Search for Meaning. Boston: Beacon Press.

76   Vollhardt, Johanna. 2009. "Altruism Born of Suffering and Prosocial Behavior Following Adverse Life Events: A Review and Conceptualization." Social Justice Research. 22: 53-97.

77   Emmons, Robert. 2007. Thanks! How the New Science of Gratitude Can Make you Happier. Boston: Houghton Mifflin.

patient is denied the opportunity to engage in a healing experience. The clinician also denies himself the benefit of engaging in the receipt of gratitude. No one would intentionally hinder the healing progress of their patients or intentionally prevent himself from being the best clinician possible, but responding this way prevents the healing capacity of giving for everyone involved. Research also suggests that if people do not donate when they think they ought to, it can lead to negative emotions like guilt and shame and to an increase in stress hormones, which negates the positive emotions and health benefits associated with philanthropic giving.[78] Ultimately, there is a cost for not engaging in charitable giving.[79]

Improved Clinical Skills

When clinicians hear and receive patients' gratitude, they also experience many benefits. Research shows when physicians experience gratitude, they are happier and more emotionally connected to their work and their patients, which results in higher patient and physician satisfaction. Happiness also makes people better complex problem solvers and, for clinicians, improves their skills as diagnosticians[80] by freeing the mind to solve problems in new and innovative ways.[81]

Engaging Physicians in the Philanthropic Process

By understanding the healing benefits of philanthropy and appreciating that a patient's donation is not a transaction but a transformational

78 Dunn, Elizabeth, Ashton-James, Clair, Hanson, Margaret, and Aknin, Lara. 2010. "On the Costs of Self-interested Economic Behavior: How Does Stinginess Get Under the Skin?" Journal of Health Psychology. 15: 627-633.

79 Schlenker, Barry. 1980. Impression management: The self-concept, social identity, and interpersonal relations. Monterey: Brooks/Cole.

80 Emmons, Robert. 2007. Thanks! How the New Science of Gratitude Can Make you Happier. Boston: Houghton Mifflin.

81 Fredrickson, Barbara. 1998. "What Good are Positive Emotions?" Review of General Psychology. 2(3): 300-316.

experience, physicians can become comfortable with their participation in the philanthropic process. To meaningfully engage physicians, leaders must operationalize a four-step program.

1. Activate Physician Champions

Hospitals and health systems need to strategically identify, recruit, train, and operationalize a system to create Physician Champions—medical partners who help the philanthropy office identify patients that are grateful, introduce those patients to the philanthropy team, and participate in the philanthropic process in a comfortable and meaningful manner.

Identifying Prospective Physician Champions

To identify prospective Physician Champions, philanthropy offices should create a list of physicians, organized by the following characteristics:

- Physicians with a wealthy panel of patients;
- Physicians who work in key service lines or centers of distinction;
- Physicians who are already active partners, as demonstrated by serving on key hospital committees, participating in special events, and donating to the organization; and
- Physicians identified by senior leaders as having a high level of emotional intelligence and receiving high patient satisfaction scores.

Physicians who are employed are generally more receptive to partnering, but those physicians who are not employed should also be given equal consideration.

Research conducted by the Gobel Group finds the ideal ratio of physician champions per philanthropy officer is 10 to one. Therefore, if a philanthropy office has four philanthropy officers, the team would want to identify 40 prospective physician champions. Once the list of prospective physician champions has been developed, it should be reviewed with the healthcare organization's chief executive officer, chief operating officer, chief medical officer, chief nursing officer, and other senior leaders. When senior leaders engage in the vetting process, they will feel ownership over the list and program.

Recruiting Physician Champions

Once your list of prospective champions is finalized, philanthropy offices will need to recruit physicians as partners. The key to recruitment is the active involvement of the healthcare organization's senior leadership. In the past, philanthropy offices would meet with physicians, explain the process, and ask for their help, and the physicians would usually agree to participate. Then nothing would happen. Meetings with the physicians would be set and then cancelled. Emails would be sent to the physicians and not returned. It's not surprising. The physicians' mindset is still based on a financial transaction, and they are not motivated to change their behavior to incorporate philanthropy into their considerations.

To successfully recruit physicians as partners in philanthropy, senior leaders must be involved. Leaders need to email or call each prospective physician champion and directly ask for that physician's help. An excellent example of a conversation between a CEO and a prospective physician champion goes like this:

"Hi, Dr. Smith. I want to tell you about a new initiative I am leading. As you know, we need to expand and diversify our revenue model, and we've identified philanthropy as a significant and untapped opportunity for growth. We know our patients are grateful for the care and compassion medical staff leaders like you are providing. So I asked my senior leadership team to help me identify a few physicians who could help us conceptualize a new program that makes it easy for patients who want to give back to contribute to your program and our hospital. I asked them to identify physicians who are or could be leaders of our institution, who are already delivering exceptional patient experiences, and who are citizens of our hospital. You were on the list. Would you join my team to help me build this program?"

Do you think Dr. Smith said no? No way. In fact, few, if any, physicians will say no to this appeal. Leveraging the influence of your CEO or other senior leader to recruit your prospective physician champions is the key.

Training Physician Champions

Once you've successfully recruited physicians to partner with your philanthropy program, the next step is getting them to think differently about the role and importance of philanthropy to the hospital or health system. Again, most physicians will think of philanthropy as a financial transaction and specifically think you want them to ask their patients for money. Even if you say that's not your plan, they will still be cautious and nervous about participating. The key is getting them to understand philanthropy is not a transaction, but a natural extension of the clinical experience they are providing to patients. When patients are grateful for the care and compassion they received, some will want to express their gratitude by giving back. Since research shows allowing patients the opportunity to give back provides health and healing benefits, why would any physician want to deny a patient an experience that can benefit their health and well-being? And you're not asking them to solicit their patients. You are just asking them to acknowledge and accept a patient's gratitude and refer them to you when the patient wants to give back.

Operationalizing Physician Engagement

While training physicians to think differently and to accept that the relationship between giving and healing is critical, it isn't enough to get physicians to act differently. To change the physician's behavior, philanthropy offices must operationalize the engagement, making it easy and efficient for the physician to partner with the philanthropy office.

The goal of this operationalization effort is to systemize the process, conceptualize collateral materials, and provide the technological tools to create grateful patient referrals. Examples of tools philanthropy offices can use to make a physician's engagement easy and efficient are:

- smartphone apps for referral of patient names,
- built-in "orders" inside an organization's EMR,
- written and video physician champion "cases for support,"
- physician web landing pages,
- philanthropy officer referral cards and posters, and
- customized letters, emails, and phone and in-person scripts for physicians to use when introducing the philanthropy officer.

2. Strengthen the Prospect Pipeline

After a hospital has identified, recruited, trained, and operationalized a physician's engagement with their philanthropy program, it will see a dramatic expansion of suspects and prospects in the development pipeline. After approximately six to twelve months of implementation, a hospital will see an average of four to six new patient names identified each month from each physician. If your philanthropy program has four philanthropy officers and 40 physicians engaged, programs can identify between 150 to 250 new suspects each month.

3. Accelerate the Productivity of the Philanthropy Team

With a more robust pipeline of prospects, philanthropy programs have the opportunity to accelerate the productivity of their philanthropy officers' activity, resulting in more visits, more asks, and more and larger gifts closed. Philanthropy officers should secure 15 or more visits each month, with most of these visits coming from prospects identified through physician referrals.

To promote acceleration, philanthropy programs should develop a personalized plan for each philanthropy officer working with each physician champion. Special training should be provided to the philanthropy officer on the best practices for partnering with physicians. Ongoing coaching and mentoring should be provided to philanthropy officers to ensure every interaction with physicians and those prospects identified is maximized.

If your philanthropy program is identifying 200 new suspects each month, you should expect approximately 25%, or in this case 50 suspects, of those names identified will be converted to a qualification visit. Therefore, each philanthropy officer can count on generating approximately 10 new qualification visits each month, using the rest of their time to manage their existing portfolio of prospects. If the philanthropy officer doesn't have time to make 10 new visits each month, the philanthropy program would just reduce the number of new suspects contacted for qualification visits.

4. Educating Hospital Employees and Creating a Culture of Gratitude

For decades, our profession has talked about the goal of creating a culture of philanthropy at hospitals. Has it happened for your hospital yet? If not, you're not alone. And it's going to be very difficult because, again, leaders, clinicians, and other hospital employees think about philanthropy as a financial transaction, not a transformative experience for patients. That's why it is essential to create a culture of gratitude. Hospital employees must understand their work creates gratitude with patients and this gratitude enables the philanthropic process to begin with patients. Everyone must know how to acknowledge and accept gratitude and, when a patient expresses an interest in giving back, how to refer that patient to the philanthropy program.

Hospital leaders talk about patient satisfaction and developing service recovery plans every day. But how much time are they spending teaching employees how to accept gratitude from patients? Not very much. Yet operationalizing a program to teach employees how to accept gratitude would not just improve patient satisfaction scores but could have a powerful impact on a patient's clinical compliance and a reduction in readmission rates, among other benefits.

Philanthropy leaders are privy to an unusually robust catalogue of positive patient stories. Deploying grateful patient stories organization-wide can reconnect the people who work in the organization to why they got into this work in the first place and keep coming to work every day. This practice reinforces an organization's values, creates meaningful and positive moments for everyone who touches the organization, introducing a palpable positive shift in the organizational culture. Simply sharing patient stories has healing capacity.[82] If you're not articulating the larger message of the power of philanthropy to heal and using these stories to create a "culture of gratitude," it's not too late to begin.

Experience has shown the effectiveness of sharing stories is through 90- to 120-second video vignettes of patients, doctors, nurses, and others talking about the healing power of philanthropy. With these vignettes, you can create powerful orientation training programs for all hospital employees, moving physician and nurse training programs, meaningful volunteer training programs, and testimonials for your websites, lobby, and in-room television networks. The use of these video vignettes to build a culture of gratitude is unlimited.

Conclusion

Without the help of physicians to identify patients who are grateful, to introduce those patients to the philanthropy team, and to be involved in the philanthropic process in a comfortable and meaningful manner, organizations deny patients the opportunity to heal. But being involved in the philanthropic process is not just for the benefit of the patients. When physicians and nurses are on the receiving end of gratitude, they become more grateful, generous, compassionate, and empathetic, engaging more fully in their work and communicating more effectively with the care team and their patients, adjusting the workplace environment. Telling these extraordinary grateful patient stories hospital-wide reconnects the entire organization with the mission of healthcare, reminding everyone of the value of their work.

Here's the bottom line. Philanthropy is not about prying money

---

82 Zak, Paul. "How Stories Change the Brain". Greater Good: The Science of Meaningful Life. Online article, December 17, 2013. Accessed February19, 2014 at http://greatergood.berkeley.edu/article/item/how_stories_change_brain.

from rich people's pockets. It's about unlocking the power of gratitude to help patients heal. When a patient is grateful for the care they have received, they are motivated to donate. When they donate and express their gratitude, they are happier. When they are happier, they can live longer lives.

Ultimately, an integrated grateful patient philanthropy program creates the environment and relationships that drive exceptional care, and ultimately more philanthropic revenue is generated for the organization. Through these additional resources, hospitals may find a pathway to support investments in the people, programs, facilities, and technology they need to create sustainable organizations in the future.

Executive Summary

- Most hospital employees today think about philanthropy as a financial transaction.
- From the patient's perspective, philanthropy is a transformational experience with the power to heal.
- Grateful patient philanthropy programs are a continuation of the clinical experience and an extension of the patient's healing journey, and they require meaningful engagement from the clinical team.
- Engaging in grateful patient philanthropy programs increases care provider engagement and satisfaction with their work and improves clinical skills, teamwork, and effectiveness in patient care.
- To meaningfully engage physicians in the philanthropic program requires training to think differently and a systemic effort to operationalize a process that makes it easy for the physician to partner with the philanthropy officer.
- Focus on creating a culture of gratitude. It drives exceptional patient care and improves the engagement and effectiveness of healthcare professionals.

Discussion

1. How are physicians engaged in your philanthropy program today?
2. Does your hospital or health system have the opportunity to grow its philanthropic revenue by meaningfully engaging more physicians in your work?
3. Will your senior leaders actively partner with you to identify and recruit prospective physician champions?
4. Do you have the resources and talent to train and operationalize a physician's engagement?
5. Are your philanthropy officers prepared to change the way they work and actively partner with physician champions to get more visits, make more asks, and close larger gifts?
6. Will your organization help you articulate the role philanthropy can play in the lives of the patients they touch?
7. What engagement, work satisfaction, teamwork, and patient communication challenges does your organization face?
8. What opportunities do you have to create a culture of gratitude at your institution?

Author Bios

Chad Gobel is founder and CEO of the Gobel Group, which specializes in engaging physicians in the philanthropic process to build grateful patient philanthropy programs. He has more than 20 years of experience in philanthropic programs, including time as Associate Chairman of Development at The Cleveland Clinic and Chief Development Officer at the University of Rochester Medical Center.

Alisa Stetzer, Senior Consultant for Strategic Research at Gobel Group, has 15 years' experience in identifying, developing, and implementing best practices in hospital clinical strategy and operations.

Fostering the Development Team
Lise Twiford, MBA, CFRE

You WORK FOR A NONPROFIT healthcare facility. You are the leader of the Development Department. The current healthcare environment is uncertain. Your CEO and the Board of Trustees are counting on philanthropic dollars to support a certain amount of the organization's expenses. You may work in a small development office or be the leader of a very large shop. Times are tough, fundraisers are in demand, and you have high financial goals. So how do you ensure the goal will be met while retaining good staff members, building a solid program, and providing a department that works in harmony? Good question! For many leaders, the answer lies in building a high-functioning team to produce exceptional results, achieve job satisfaction, invite an environment of open communication, and overcome pervasive employee turnover.

A well-rounded development office is not hard to produce when given the backing and approval of the administration and the Board of Directors. If you are in a situation where organizational leadership does not understand or embrace development, you may not be on the right bus to accomplish your own personal or professional goals or to galvanize a strong team. If, however, you are fortunate enough to work for an organization that knows or is willing to learn the value of philanthropy, the next step is to create a dynamic team that is willing to stay for the long haul. This ultimate challenge merits intent to accomplish.

Leadership

In his book, *The 21 Irrefutable Laws of Leadership*, John C. Maxwell states that leadership is influence—nothing more, nothing less. Harry A. Overstreet, a popular lecturer and author on modern psychology and sociology, notes that the very essence of the power to influence lies in getting the other person to participate. That said, the chief development officer (CDO), and all frontline fundraisers (many of whom will be future leaders) must have and develop their circle of influence. By working daily with prospects, donors, and leadership—both internal and external to the community—this builds influence by leveraging participation though charitable giving, volunteering, and spreading goodwill.

Developing influence, however, is not achieved simply by gaining a title; rather, it is developed over time with consistent and diligent work. Training and preparation are continuous activities in the life of a leader. Boxer Joe Fraizer stated, "You can map out a fight plan or a life plan, but when the action starts, you're down to your reflexes. That's where your road work shows. If you cheated on that in the dark of the morning, you're getting found out now under the bright lights" ("The Champ," *Reader's Digest*, January 1972, 109). If you are in a position of leadership or considering climbing the corporate ladder, you must be willing to maintain a lifetime of continual professional learning.

Once you have committed to continually honing your leadership skills, you now have the task of effectively managing the development team. Hiring new staff may be necessary, but you may already have a team in place that has a long history with the organization. Now is the time to evaluate the team and set the stage for success. If you are a leader who has been with the organization and you have a long history with the department, it is imperative that you reevaluate your team on an annual basis to ensure ongoing effectiveness. You should also see who is excelling and take the opportunity to help those individuals advance their careers. In other words, do not take anyone or any successful program for granted. Plants need water, and as they grow, they often need to be repotted to expand their roots. A great leader is a great gardener.

Evaluating your team and the functions they perform takes a concerted effort. First, take stock of who is sitting on your development-office bus. Do they have the right skills? How did they get there? What are their personal goals and expectations? The team is the most important part of a successful development program. As a leader, you must evaluate each team member for skills and willingness to be a team player. Establishing this understanding takes an exceptional amount of communication—the kind few leaders are willing to embrace. Why? It is hard and can be exhausting to truly listen to insights, criticisms, perceptions, and expectations about the organization, the team members' colleagues, and you as a leader. It is difficult to determine if your staff members are on the right seat on the bus. Are you willing to embrace an open environment and hear how your colleagues and you, personally, are perceived? Some of those perceptions may be accurate, some may be contrived, but standing before your truth is a humbling and emancipating endeavor that will either build trust with your team or underscore their feelings and perceptions.

Once you have taken stock of your staff (and of yourself), it's time to lay the pieces on the table and make sure each member of the team has the skills needed to fulfill his or her goals. After your evaluation and conversations, you are likely to find staff in roles for which they are not well suited or do not have the proper skills. In these instances, they may need assistance finding a better fit in your office or organization, or they may be better suited leaving to join another organization. This is not be an easy discussion, but it will be one that ultimately benefits both parties when handled with respect. You will also find staff members who are highly qualified and in the perfect position. These staff members need all the support, training, and flexibility you can give them to keep them working at the top of their license. Don't take them for granted. These top fundraisers are highly sought after by other organizations and are not easily replaced, particularly when they have built relationships with your donors, leadership, and community.

It is important to understand the high cost of employee turnover, since the average amount of time a fundraiser stays at his or her job has dropped from 18 months to 16 months. This extraordinarily high turn-over of fundraisers is costing charities money—lots of money. Direct and indirect costs of finding a replacement are nearly $130,000. Below is a list of additional, real costs to the organization that can reach 150% of the employee's annual compensation figure. For managerial and frontline fundraisers, the cost can be significantly higher: reaching 200% to 250% of the annual compensation (William G. Bliss, President of Bliss & Associates Inc.). Some of the direct and indirect costs to consider include:

- Person(s) who fill(s) in while the position is vacant;
- Lost productivity at a minimum of 50% of the person's compensation and benefits for each week the position is vacant (100% if vacant for a long period of time);
- Time to conduct an exit interview;
- Administration to stop payroll, benefit deductions, benefit enrollments, and COBRA notification and administration;
- Manager who has to understand what work remains and how to cover the work until a replacement if found;
- Training, licensure, academic education, etc. that your organization has invested in the departing employee;
- Impact on departmental productivity because the person is leaving;
- Severance and benefits continuation for eligible employees;
- Lost knowledge, skills, and contacts the person who is leaving takes with him or her;
- Unemployment insurance premiums;
- Losing donor loyalty and confidence in the organization;
- Recruitment, including advertising (classified ads can run into the thousands of dollars);
- Internal recruiter or manager's time to evaluate potential candidates (ranging from 30 to over 100 hours per person);
- Background and reference checks;

- Candidate pre-employment tests to assess skills, abilities, aptitude, attitude, values, and behaviors;
- Orientation to the organization, the department, and the position;
- Person(s) time in conducting the training;
- Supplying new equipment and technology germane to the position;
- Supervisory time (and lost productivity) spent in assigning, explaining, and reviewing work assignments and output;
- Mistakes the new employee makes during the indoctrination period; and
- Intake procedures such as putting the person on payroll, establishing computer and security passwords, business cards, internal and external publicity announcements (when appropriate), telephone hookups, establishing credit card accounts, and procuring other equipment including computer tablets, pagers, and cell phones.

Beyond the financial costs to replace a position, there is an even greater cost: the time it takes to rebuild donor trust and establish new bonds when you rehire. This can take years and set your development program back significantly.

According to Penelope Burk, president of Cygnus Applied Research, there are two key reasons people leave:

- To get a better salary (only 21% of chief executives said they were in a position to offer salaries that were competitive) and
- To secure a more senior position because the institution does not provide a structure for advancement.

Developing a structure of advancement within the development office has always been problematic, given the specificity of skills required for each area of fundraising. That said, if an employee wishes to learn another role so she can advance while maintaining personal productivity, it is imperative that a savvy leader provide the opportunity, mentoring, and training for her to do so. Succession planning and training employees who want to rise to the next level will provide a win-win situation for the employee, the organization, the donor community, and you. The cost of training and mentoring is far less than the cost of employee turnover.

Wise organizations will understand the revenue-generating purpose of the department and ensure there are enough frontline fundraisers and support staff to allow for as much productivity as possible.

There is a need to be sensitive to the often understated value of support staff. Even in a lean environment, a productive ratio of frontline fundraisers to support staff must be maintained. With appropriate support, revenue-producing staff can remain focused solely on raising funds. Too often, development organizations take support staff for granted. However, when revenue-generating professionals are not in the office, the support staff answers the phone, talks with donors, and ensures gifts are properly recorded and acknowledged. Do not underestimate the value and ability of your support staff to help build and maintain a positive donor experience.

Career Mentoring

Career mentoring is an important part of fostering the development team. Do not wait until the employee comes to ask about career growth. Rather, make this an annual or semi-annual discussion with staff members. Getting this focused attention may be a surprise to some staff members, as they may not expect that anyone would want to see them move forward. On the other hand, some individuals may be completely content in their roles and do not want to move forward. That said, the only way you will determine the career aspirations of the team is to have direct, one-on-one conversations. For those who are hungry to grow, do everything possible to help define their current strengths, meet their goals, and find a position within your shop for them to move up to when the time is right.

Depth and Breadth of Development—Office Staff

While depth and breadth of staff size differ from organization to organization, there are key positions that must be included in the development program. With the support of key leadership, the organizational chart of the development staff should include personnel to cover each area of fundraising, including special events, annual giving, grants, major and planned gifts, database management, and gift processing. If possible, a prospect researcher is a plus. In small shops, functions are often combined; for example, special events and annual giving may be accomplished by hiring one or two people. Smaller shops may need to outsource functions such as grant writing and planned giving. In larger shops, there may be numerous staff members working in one area; for example, a major gift shop can range from 5 to more than 100, depending on the organization's structure. The number of staff for each development activity is dependent on whether it is a stand-alone hospital, a network of several hospitals, or a regional facility with multiple campuses. Regardless of the size of the staff or their location, leadership and team communication is imperative if fundraising efforts are to be efficient and highly successful.

Communication and career opportunity are significant drivers in either reducing or driving turnover rates. Providing an environment of open communication and strategically working with your staff on career advancement takes a strong commitment by the CDO. The CDO must not only be a well-rounded professional with extensive experience in all areas of fundraising and development but also one who is open to sharing his or her knowledge and skills to assist each director and manager in the department. The larger the size of the shop, the more difficult the task will be. Developing a culture of communication and career growth cannot be accomplished in a vacuum. The human resources department, organizational effectiveness department, or outside consultants can assist in training and coaching supervisory staff to enhance management skills. If the development leader lacks these skills himself but is truly interested in creating a motivated and satisfied team, then he must take the lead, get training, and be the model for change. Leaders should also not hesitate to share their own weaknesses and show their willingness to improve; doing so builds trust.

Office Dynamics

Raising funds for an organization is not rocket science. It is, however, very hard work that requires an immense amount of collaboration. As with most businesses, office politics and team dynamics can become a tremendous stumbling block if not kept in check. Each member of the team brings a personality and attitudes that were created as a result of his or her upbringing, culture, and life experiences. When hiring staff, it is tremendously important to have the entire team meet and have conversations with the potential candidate. "Fit" is everything. Even then, one may discover a misfit. This is where a solid 30-, 60-, and 90-day review process is key. Within the first 30 to 90 days, leaders will have the opportunity to determine a new team member's true skills, receive staff feedback, and determine if he will be an effective team player. If not, do not hesitate to end the relationship before a toxic environment can evolve. Regardless of efforts to maintain a positive, functional team, there will be a continual ebb and flow of collegiality, fun, moodiness, passive-aggressive behavior, collaboration, withholding, unsupportive cliques, undermining activities, celebrations, and dissention. This human factor is to be expected.

There will be days when a seemingly large portion of time is spent dealing with issues revolving around personalities and the struggle to get along and move in unison. To believe harmony will be the norm is to believe in Nirvana, where everyone will act as mature adults and all work together for a common goal. But negative office dynamics are extraordinarily toxic. The leader must have a keen sense of when tensions are rising and address the issue immediately. The goal is to keep negativity at a minimum by taking the office pulse regularly and putting out the sparks before they begin to flame.

Waiting until you have time only makes the issues fester and the repair process take much longer, and this challenge is one that can cause your staff to become miserable, feel unsupported, and potentially look for a position elsewhere. This means turnover that leads to lost time and revenue and a poorly functioning team. Address the issues head-on. Be an outstanding listener, take the actions you say you will, and remember you can't please everyone.

Training, Education, and Honing Skills

Fostering a development team includes providing each member with a clear understanding and expectation of his or her role. Of course, the hiring process is where the stage is set for expectations of the position. In development, however, it is very difficult to find individuals who purposefully went to school seeking a career in nonprofit fundraising. Additionally, many on the team have simply been placed into the role as a matter of necessity by the organization's leadership. That said, training is everything to set individual staff members up for success. Conferences, webinars, and professional books are wonderful for learning new techniques and networking with others; but nothing takes the place of in-house one-on-one and group training.

As you plan strategic training sessions, it is very valuable to include your staff in creating the training. Otherwise, you may make incorrect assumptions about the skills that need to be addressed and how to provide them. If you stop and truly listen to the team, you will learn exactly where they are stumbling. Together, you can create a method of training that accomplishes what they need. Then continue to discuss ways of enhancing education by providing sessions more often or including additional staff, such as annual giving and special events. The priorities, frequency, topics, and delivery methods will vary from shop to shop, but the collaboration and gratification of the endeavor will bring big returns.

Intelligence Quotient, Emotional Intelligence, and Poise

As noted above, each member of the development team has his own personality, strengths, and weaknesses. Leaders must evaluate the team and determine how effective each person is in his role and if there are opportunities for advancement or areas that need work. Does he have the appropriate intellect for the position he holds? This will most certainly differ depending on the type of work being done. However, let's explore the desired and necessary skills of frontline fundraisers.

Frontline fundraisers include revenue-generating specialists in annual giving, special events, major gifts, planned giving, grants, and stewardship. In small shops, many of these specialties are handled by one or a few people. In larger shops, each area of specialization is filled by one or many individuals doing the same or similar tasks. Regardless of staff size, frontline fundraisers must possess both academic and emotional intelligence as well as poise, confidence, and flexibility to meet and speak professionally with a wide variety of people. Finding people who possess these qualities is difficult at best. This ability to meet people where they are is not a quality that is easily found or taught. It is imperative for frontline fundraisers to be capable of one day comfortably meeting with a CEO of a major corporation who sits behind a five-foot-wide, mahogany desk and meet the next day with a donor who has the equivalent of a 1940 schoolroom desk. Flexibility to relate to people from all economic backgrounds is a critical skill. To effectively listen to the prospect/donor and be nimble enough to switch gears regarding the level of formality, tone, and physical stance is the difference between a fair to poor frontline fundraiser and an outstanding frontline fundraiser.

There is a theory that all frontline fundraisers and particularly CDOs must have *gravitas* as a primary quality in order to fulfill their role effectively. *Gravitas* defined includes descriptors such as seriousness, lordliness, somber, dignified, of importance, and the center of gravity. If the theory were fully sound, frontline fundraisers would be effective only occasionally. What is under consideration here is the absolute need to be agile in knowing the appropriate demeanor required to be with donors from all walks of life. This requires a high level of emotional intelligence. To be in *gravitas* mode while sitting with a donor who is looking for someone who laughs, listens to jokes, and has fun in life would be like rain pouring down at a Fourth of July fireworks event. Emotional intelligence comes into play when frontline fundraisers knows when to be serious and somber and when to let their hair down a bit. The reverse is also true. It is important to know when you are sitting in front of someone who views himself as the center of gravity (the ultimate *gravitas*), and you can bring your demeanor to the level of the donor. It is also critical to know that in any circumstance when politics, religion, and cultural attitudes are being shared, the savvy fundraiser will just listen and nod.

Executive Summary

- Fostering the development team takes time, patience, superb listening skills, and the ability to balance work and administration. It also takes a sincere desire to assist your staff in moving their careers forward (if that is their desire), providing educational opportunities as your budget allows, being inclusive and transparent when appropriate, knowing you will never satisfy everyone, as well as striving to keep everyone working at the top of their license and as a team to meet both individual and group goals. All these are more easily said than accomplished.
- Sincere leadership that provides each staff member with the best opportunities possible takes work. Not all of your good intensions will be realized. If you work with a small shop, you may have greater influence but fewer resources to maximize your staff's desire to grow. If you work with a larger shop, you will most certainly face challenges such

as changes in HR policies, your ability to add staff, and budget cuts.

- The smart, caring leader will find ways to keep the team educated, cohesive, and productive. Fundraising and development takes creative thought. This creativity must be applied to retaining, educating, rewarding and motivating staff. If your staff is nurtured, they will work hard, feel compelled to attain personal and group goals, and work collaboratively to ensure success. Ultimately, turnover will be limited and funds raised will increase.

Discussion:

1. How can you cultivate your own authentic leadership style?
2. How can you create a stronger and more effective team to advance the vision and mission of your organization?
3. What impediments keep you from delivering the level of collaboration and performance that are possible?
4. How can you enhance your selection process to ensure new members of the team have the skills, abilities, and qualities to advance your work?

Author Bio

Lise Twiford is vice president of development at Lehigh Valley Hospital and Health Network in Allentown, Pennsylvania.

Special Leadership Topics

The Strategic Value of Centralized Business Services to the Multi-System Philanthropic Enterprise

Jay Maloney, CFRE

THERE IS STRATEGIC IMPORTANCE to standardizing the business services of integrated, multi-system fundraising programs. This chapter will guide you not so much on *how* to do it but on *why* to do it. The discussion will be presented from a strategic mindset, and while the conversation is relevant to any system of any size, this chapter is oriented toward larger, complex systems.

You will progress through a number of things here. The things for you to keep in mind are that human nature of real people living in the real world will always trump organization charts, and the laws of unintended consequences always come into play at the most unexpected times. The case to create a central, standardized business-services operation is real and compelling. Threading your way through human nature is the challenge.

Integrated health systems generally come into being by slowly and gradually coming together. Over time they can become quite large. The case example system here, Catholic Health Initiatives (CHI), is one of the nation's largest, stretching from coast to coast and border to border, across all four time zones, with more than 90 facilities in 19 states. Within CHI, there are 72 development programs or foundations. CHI's entire network of foundations share centrally managed business services out of the system's Colorado Springs-based support center. The support center employs about 40 people. The operation maintains more than 1.6 million records. The organization processes more than a half-million gifts each year. It supports 25,000 projects each year (big and small, scheduled and stat). It produces more than 100 major mail efforts annually. The work done is sent to each foundation, so it always appears to be local. The final owner of projects for each foundation is also the local development leader. The CHI foundations' support system was built in phases over 30 years.

Business Support is a Strategic Issue, Not an Operational Issue

There is power to integrating a network of disparate development programs into a coherent force. Everyone sees the value of standardizing best practices into their system. Yet many systems—perhaps most of them—find themselves tied in knots when they set off to build the thing.

The root of their frustrations has less to do with the architecture of how they will integrate their fundraising programs than with their potential failure to grasp the *strategic importance* of integrating the business systems that support the organization's efforts.

Many organizations view the idea of "centralized backroom services" as simply a route to more cost savings. Cost savings are important, but focusing solely on cost savings is too narrow an objective. It is a *finance* mindset that sadly comes to dominate the bigger *enterprise* mindset.

The context of the philanthropic enterprise is all about relationships. It is not about transactions. To create a business support center for a foundation that focuses solely on transaction management is to completely misunderstand the nature of the philanthropic enterprise.

The philanthropic enterprise is quite different from the healthcare enterprise. The business systems that support the healthcare enterprise are not optimal (and sometimes not even functional) to support the philanthropic enterprise.

Opportunities emerge when a system decides to integrate its development programs through system-wide business services. A good support system does not create a one-size-fits-all bureaucracy but should allow for each program to exercise its own personality and its own signature activities.

A consolidated, or centralized, foundation support system should be able to do the following things for all of the system's development programs whether they are large or small, whether they have tens of employees or fewer than a single employee.

- **Reduce the high cost of redundant data-processing systems.** A single, integrated business system can re-code all of the varying information systems into a standardized and uniformly coded set of databases, or into a sophisticated customer relationship management (CRM) system. An integrated system can secure and share discount pricing on products from key vendors through a potential partnership with those vendors.

- **Mitigate or eliminate the spotty quality of major gift activity across the system (and too many financially underachieving fundraising events).** A central support system can minimize many of the administrative tasks that keep development professionals in the office. The central support system can relieve more time to spend on activities that generate fundraising revenues. It can also minimize event or project activities that are generally time-intensive, high-cost, and low return on investment (ROI).

- **Eliminate inaccurate, inconsistent, and untimely information.** A central support system, employing well-trained and well-managed operators, can update records and maintain the quality and integrity of donors' sensitive records. This stable, centrally managed team will also protect the integrity of the coding structures. They can run queries, lists, mailings, and reports when they are needed with just-in-time data. Under the guidance of a centralized management process, they can provide standard or specialized coding for all of the development programs.

- **Create uniformly managed data-processing competency among all employees.** A central support function can reformat all of the disparate database coding into a uniform and long-term information language. This eliminates the habits and outcomes of *ad hoc* coding that typically result from (and are subject to) local employee turnover. This stable body of employees ensures data integrity across the system. It also ensures a consistent, institutional memory.

- **Ensure predictable communication and coordination among the local health system foundations.** A central support system can manage and coordinate all projects throughout the system through a centralized calendar. This allows for coordinated mailings with materials that are purchased and produced toward greater economies of scale and cost savings. The centralized system provides for a "central nervous system" repository for all development activity taking place across a system.

- **Eliminate untimely and disparate financial management systems.** A centralized support system results in streamlined and uniform gift processing process. Specialists at the system level can review gift processing batches for accounting accuracy to minimize accounting and acknowledgement mistakes. Staff can also provide standardized, consistent financial reporting that allows the system to set benchmarks and create measurable future goals.

So Why Isn't This Easy to Do?

Let's set those important and desirable things aside for a while and return to the discussion on how and why systems find themselves tied in knots.

Consider this common visual image that you have likely seen in one form or another. It sometimes involves an illustration of a stick figure or two standing at the upper left side (usually defined as *today* or *present stable state*). The figures are getting ready for a journey over to the upper right side of the slide (usually defined as *tomorrow* or *future stable state*). Exhibit 1 displays an example of this visual.

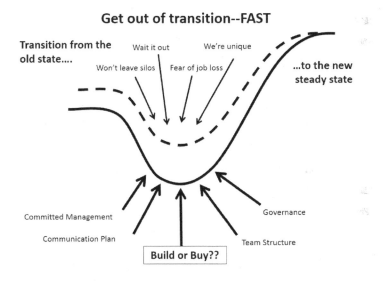

There's a U-shaped gap placed between the present and future states. Sometimes it is displayed as a valley or a depression.

The *y*-axis (the one that goes up and down) is usually presented as a representation of good things such as *quality, efficiency,* or *customer satisfaction*. Being up on this chart is good, while being down is not good.

The *x*-axis (the one that goes left to right) is usually presented as *time*.

The *future stable state* located at the upper right side of that U-curve is always illustrated as being a bit higher on the *y*-axis than is the *present stable state*. What this means, of course, is that the future stable state—the "new order"—promises to be better than the present state. The gap or valley informs us the transition from one state to the other will create some period in which things you presently do well will deteriorate for a while until you get yourself to the new and better state. This deterioration of quality is a given during any transition, whether the transition is brief or lengthy.

There are a few critical elements to all this imagery. One of them is the *x*-axis—*time*. Time is the enemy. The longer any transition period goes on, the more difficult it becomes to get to that promised new state. If the transition drags on and the quality of your business remains deteriorated for too long, the pressures to abandon the venture become greater and greater.

For system-level development leaders who are charged with integrating a variety of development programs into some sort of effective whole, the dynamic of downward pressures at the *y*-axis, and the lengthening forces at the *x*-axis come alive *as soon as you begin discussing the integration process.*

The good news is there are also some upward and supporting pressures found along *x*. These upward pressures are finite, political, and shorter-lived than the downward pressures.

Lengthy transition is a strategic risk. What the graphic cannot show you fully is the deterioration of the quality of work, while a very significant factor, is not as corrosive as is the length of time the quality stays down. Therefore, it is vital that you move from the old state to the new state in as short a time as possible.

In the case of building a unifying fundraising enterprise for a health system, installing standardized business services is the single greatest contributor to lengthy transition time. Yet integrated business systems are frequently the last thing development leaders attend to. Worse, the failure to install a standardized system in a timely way serves to strengthen the downward forces and weaken the upward forces.

So just what are these upward and downward forces? From where do they come and how to they affect your strategy?

Let's begin with some of the upward, positive forces. Almost always, the upward forces are the more intellectual and rational reasons to integrate. Some examples of upward forces include:

- the list of desirable outcomes described above
- a committed board or governing body
- committed senior leadership
- a solid communications plan that describes the mission and financial value of the integration
- the organizational design and business plan that defines the future state
- your personal commitment and leadership

The downward forces are less intellectual, less rational, and elemental to human nature itself. These downward forces are contributors to but not the cause of lengthy and difficult transitions. They are generally highly emotional and personal in nature, and they feel closer to home, as far as the affected employees are concerned. With few exceptions, they are not at all the result of malicious intent, and they are not aimed at disrupting anything. They are simply a display of human nature.

These downward forces have an advantage over the upward forces. The upward forces generally do not increase as additional players are added to the formula, and the upward forces tend to fatigue over time. However, the more organizations you bring together, the weightier and more complex the downward pressures become, and the downward forces also tend to grow in strength over time.

Some examples of downward forces that keep quality lower than it needs to be for longer than it needs to be include the following:

- employees across the foundation network who know how to wait things out ("This is management's impulse of the week. It too will pass.")
- employees who fear job change or loss
- employees (and volunteers) steeped in silo thinking, silo habits, and silo politics
- belief that "our community is different"

With all that said, a working and sea-tested, integrated business-support system has to transition from its present-state silos into its future-state system and do it FAST.

Without an integrated business system in place, your fundraising programs will never quite mesh. As time ticks by, the support from beneath to integrate the fundraising programs begins to wane. The upward support from leadership begins to conclude there is *something* about your particular fundraising system that just will not or cannot accommodate integration. The *something* that governance and senior leadership senses to be amiss is not the development programs.

Likely, in fact, the development programs have a fair number of things in common that can and should accommodate a move to system-ness. Rather, the problematic *something* is more often than not a disorganized family of development-office business practices that are wildly incompatible with one another. As mentioned earlier, integrated health systems generally come into being slowly and gradually. Each organization brings with it decades of habits, values, rituals, and processes that color and shade the entity-development program. Each market-based development program has lived with its own procedures and practices, its own information system code structures, and its own vocabulary. Each is plugged into a hospital or health system finance department that digests and processes development program numbers in its own special way. All in all, it is here on the business side of things where you find the core of your challenges.

In larger systems where there are many development programs involved, this variety of business systems creates a truly intractable problem for the upward forces to overcome—and a hidden blessing for the downward forces to enjoy. (Recall the downward forces can multiply their effects almost exponentially, the more programs that are involved.)

Senior development leadership at the system level can unwittingly become a part of this downward dynamic and even add to it. Development executives in large organizations focus their thinking on *fundraising* systems. They correctly and capably focus their energies on things such as prospect management, sales-team management, pipeline management, and so on. They are generally not attuned to the business-support systems that operate in the background. They tend to delegate this important element of their work to skilled and talented lieutenants.

Whether a development program is large or small, each has its own culture, with particular habits, values, and ways of doing things. It also has its own language. One reason why it is so challenging to integrate development programs into the system is they each have their own vocabulary. A *major gift* in one place is most likely not the same thing as a *major gift* in another place. The health system must adopt a common language if it is to succeed in building an integrated fundraising system. One of the important elements of an organization's internal language is found within the code structure of its information system. This is especially true for development programs.

For instance, assume for discussion's sake that the development programs in a system all use the same donor-management software. You will likely discover each software program has been around for a while and each program is coded very differently. You will likely also discover that coding at some, many, or all development programs has not been diligently maintained and that different staff members have independently added codes or made entry decisions unbeknownst to management.

Let's also assume there are two or more programs that have (or believe themselves to have) solid and well-built "backroom services." Each is convinced its support system should become the system's sole surviving system and organizational standard. Here again, you bump into human nature.

Learning Curves (and the Law of Unintended Consequences)

You owe it to yourself (and your organization) to acknowledge right up front that all of the best, well-considered plans and schemes are subject to the least-discussed variable in business: The Law of Unintended Consequences.

The Law of Unintended Consequences has been around in one form or another since the days of philosopher and economist Adam Smith.

More recently, it has come to be used as a short, memorable warning that intervention into any complex system tends to create unanticipated (and occasionally undesirable) outcomes. Many people compare it to Murphy's Law, which says, "Anything that can go wrong will go wrong." It is a real and serious thing, yet it is commonly used as a humorous warning against the self-confident and self-centered belief that humans can fully control the world around us. Big organizations of all stripes fit into this definition.

In his 1936 paper, *"On Social Structure and Science,"* sociologist Robert Merton described five possible causes of what he called "unanticipated consequences":

- *Ignorance*—It is impossible to anticipate everything, thereby leading to incomplete analysis;
- *Error*—Incorrect analysis of the problem or the following of habits that worked in the past but may not apply to the current situation;
- *Short-term interest*—which may override long-term interests;
- *Conflicting Basic Values*—where certain actions may be either required or prohibited, even if their long-term result might be unfavorable; and
- *Self-defeating* or *self-fulfilling prophecies*—where the fear of some consequence drives people to do negative things before the feared problem ever occurs.

Recall that the decision to build—or to buy—centralized business services is a *strategic* decision. In all likelihood, your integrated development programs will never assimilate without centralized business services. The *build* decision involves many things, such as workflow analysis at each site, review and analysis of each contender's coding structures, and staffing decisions regarding talent you currently employ versus the talent that you will need to recruit. There will be decisions to make regarding physical location of the business support center, which will affect your talent decisions. However, if you do not have the time, risk capacity, or resources to build the business support system, you could alternatively buy such services from a provider who has already navigated the issues at hand.

While it is true that centralized business support will standardize your foundation's transactions, the nature of the service is not transactional. The fund development profession is relationship-driven by nature. Every major gift prospect is a unique individual. There are nuances to each relationship that demand a support system that will accommodate enormous degrees of customization. Support staff must be intimately engaged with prospect-by-prospect work of the development officers. The same degree of attention must be given to the complex lists and campaigns designed by the annual gifts team. Failure to do that reflects directly and terribly on the fundraisers. However, effectively deploying a centralized business-services effort can and will have positive, strategic implications that can enable you to achieve more than you ever could without such a commmon language and platform.

Executive Summary

- Large health systems grow through steady and occasionally sudden progression in coming together. The fundraising programs within a system come from many cultures and habits. Each has its own management languages ranging from definition of terms, to preferred fundraising doctrine, to the coding within their databases. *Until the system standardizes those elemental things, the integrated development system will never quite take off.*

- To standardize the processes and performance expectations of the system's disparate development programs, a centralized and unifying business-support center is needed. *The time necessary to install such a centralized support center frequently takes longer than the time granted by leadership to get it done.*

- *Human nature* (fear of change, fear of job loss, silo mentality, or wait-it-out attitude) plus the *Law of Unintended Consequences* (failure to anticipate events that become a chain of events, erroneous starting assumptions, or not knowing all the factors) conspire to drag out conversions of silos into standardized systems. To attenuate those two conspiring factors, you could consider buying the service from a service partner rather than building the service on your own.

Discussion

1. Do the fundraising programs in your system have an established set of guiding principles from which they design and carry out their programs (*i.e.*, ROI is a key driver, sales is the key culture, major gifts are elemental to success, activity and results are measured uniformly, etc.)?
2. Does your system define production and effort uniformly, across all development programs? And are you fully comfortable that the numbers (and definitions) of production and effort are computed uniformly across the board?
3. Are your foundations able to focus maximum time and energy on major gift investors rather than on large numbers of smaller donors (more time with better prospects)?
4. Do you have a high level of faith in the quality of the information that you use to make decisions, and do you have a high level of faith that all foundations are counting/reporting apples to apples?
5. Do your foundations fully understand and can they articulate the system story as an element of their own local story, one that enriches and expands the local story?

Author Bio

Joseph V. "Jay" Maloney is president and chief executive officer of the Catholic Health Initiatives Foundation. He previously served as a foundation executive with Centura Health, Englewood, CO, and was previously with CHI and one of its predecessor organizations, Sisters of Charity Health Care System, for almost 25 years.

The Campaign Mix:
The 5 P's of Successful
Hospital Capital Campaigning

William J. Mountcastle

THE MARKETING MIX is a well-known business tool used by marketing professionals. The term was first used and popularized in the late 1940s by Neil H. Borden of Harvard Business School when he authored "The Concept of the Marketing Mix." According to Borden, he got the inspiration for the term from his colleague James Culliton. Culliton first described the "mixer of ingredients": one who sometimes follows recipes prepared by others, sometimes prepares his own recipe as he goes along, and sometimes adapts a recipe from immediately available ingredients. Culliton brought to light the essential ingredients, all beginning with the letter *P*: product, placement, price, and promotion. A fifth ingredient, people, was added later. These 5 *P*'s are a set of controllable variables, often regarded as the core of any marketing system. They are considered universal, timeless, and essential truths in marketing.

The Marketing Mix can be adapted to create the Campaign Mix that drives inspired fund development campaigns through the 5 *P*'s of successful capital campaigning. Like the Marketing Mix, these ingredients are timeless and should be seen as the core of a campaign.

The five essential ingredients are:
- Preparation,
- People,
- Pervasiveness,
- Passion, and
- Persistence.

These ingredients, when carefully mixed together and balanced, are the perfect recipe for a successful hospital capital campaign.

Preparation

Not unlike the Boy Scouts, hospitals should be properly prepared before entering a fundraising campaign. The Boy Scouts teach preparedness by encouraging scouts to think out beforehand any situation that might occur, so one might recognize the right thing to do at the right moment and be willing to do it. Campaign preparation can take months, or even years, and involve dozens of people. A carefully organized approach will help lead to a successful conclusion.

1. Align with the Hospital's Strategic Plan

Any discussion of a campaign should start with the strategic planning process. Best-practice hospitals use research-driven analysis and tested planning approaches to evaluate their market, provide a road map, and set future-focused goals. In relation to fundraising, there are three undeniable propositions in hospital strategic planning: 1) the dynamics of the new healthcare environment have magnified expectations to realize more consistent, predictable philanthropic revenue to offset growing pressure on hospital operating margins, 2) philanthropy is now an increasingly valuable revenue source for funding hospitals' future strategic investments, and 3) a hospital's operational and fundraising success depends on a collaborative alignment between the two. There should be no disconnect between the hospital's operations and its fundraising, especially when preparing for a campaign. The hospital's board, executive leadership, and fundraising office must together evaluate needs for programs and services. Plan objectives should be based on valuable and legitimate institutional plans, goals, budgets, and needs. Most hospital strategic plans share ambitions to become leaders in the industry, attract high-quality staff and health experts, and establish cutting-edge services for their communities. With these aims, successful hospitals achieve short- and long-term growth through the constant evaluation of future-focused operational and financial goals.

The proposed programs and projects that require community philanthropy should be driven by community and program needs and be consistent with the overall strategic plan. However, under no circumstances should a hospital's ability to raise money in a campaign dictate the strategic direction a hospital advances, or as commonly said, "The tail should not be wagging the dog." Campaign fundraising must be in furtherance of the hospital's goals, rather than the reverse. It can be easy for fundraising offices to be tempted to put forward a strategic suggestion for the hospital because it is popular with a key donor or group of donors, even if it isn't fully consistent with the hospital's mission and values. Yes, it may be difficult to refuse would-be opportunities when funding is tight or goals are great; but the hospital exists to serve a mission, and the strategic plan dictates how to get there. The mission must be front and center in determining opportunities to pursue or tactics to pursue them—in fundraising just as much as in strategic direction.

2. Explore Opportunities Beyond Bricks and Mortar

Hospital priorities are shifting away from traditional bricks-and-mortar projects because hospital leaders are starting to question whether they should be raising millions of dollars for physical expansion rather than for projects that could expand capacity in other, even better, ways. In recent years, campaigns have been used to fund a wide variety of special projects intended to enable an organization to serve more people and have greater impact on the community. Beyond the bricks and mortar, fundraisers might ask campaign donors to invest in aligning processes and development of better care coordination between hospital and ambulatory providers to ensure seamless care, retaining and recruiting physicians, promoting evidence-based practices to improve quality and patient safety, advancing disease management programs and prevention initiatives, and improving efficiency through productivity and financial management. Leaders increasingly are looking for ways to cut redundant efforts and standardize processes to cut costs and improve patient care, and future campaigns should support such efforts.

Modern hospital capital investment needs are increasingly technology-related. Organizations are increasingly seeking philanthropy to improve technology and computerized tracking systems to increase patient flow, integrate information systems to improve patient care, and invest in sophisticated data mining and analysis. Development offices will raise money for these organization-building technologies because they will strengthen our hospitals and allow them to achieve more mission impact, more effectively.

3. Establish the Length and Scope of the Effort

A campaign is a defining moment in the life of any nonprofit hospital, so establishing the length and scope of a campaign is an essential part of campaign preparation. Today hospitals need to think through whether to move forward with a:

- Traditional campaign: a time-limited effort to raise significant dollars, often to fund construction or renovation of a building;
- Mini-campaign: a condensed, focused effort that targets smaller groups of individuals for specific objectives; or a
- Perpetual campaign: a no-end campaign, or an ongoing journey for which campaign completion is not the final destination.

Some maintain traditional, comprehensive capital campaigns are the only way to do campaigning. Others say traditional campaigns are a thing of the past because they are not agile and cannot anticipate and absorb changes in funding priorities and volunteer commitments. Still others argue the future is the perpetual campaign, in which the organization is continuously in campaign mode: either preparing for a campaign, in one, or getting ready for the next one. Each has both positive and negative implications that must be considered and managed. To determine a campaign's length and scope, organizations should evaluate:

- Revenue needed,
- Health of the existing prospect pipeline, and
- Engagement of hospital staff and volunteers.

In any case, utilize the campaign as a vehicle for asking for bigger gifts, getting in front of the community, and energizing the board and leadership volunteers to be future-focused.

4. Conduct a Feasibility Study

Conducting a feasibility study is an absolutely essential step in campaign preparation. Most hire a consulting firm to conduct a study, but this is not always the case. The principal value of hiring a firm is that community leaders, physicians, grateful patients, and donors who are interviewed for the study will often be more comfortable and forthright in talking with an "objective third party" than with a hospital staff member. A good study will assess the likelihood of success for a campaign, identify strategies and specific individual givers, determine how the hospital is viewed in the eyes of prospective donors, determine the community's understanding of the importance of the proposed investments, determine whether the hospital has access to financial resources sufficient to reach its campaign goal, assess hospital infrastructure and ability to handle all particulars of a campaign, and help set a realistic campaign goal and timeline.

5. Create a Captivating Case for Support

Once a hospital has conducted a feasibility study, the next step is to develop a case for support. Successful campaigning is founded on making a strong case that builds upon the feasibility study research to articulate what most excites donors about the campaign. When a hospital's case is clear and focused, its fundraising dollars increase substantially. The case must effectively tell your hospital story and convey key messages, as well as describe how the campaign will make a difference. It is important to position the case from the donor's point of view rather than the hospital's need.

In addition to the full case statement, organizations should create an elevator pitch that provides a set of short and snappy talking points for the campaign. These talking points are used by hospital and volunteer leaders and fundraising staff to succinctly lay out the importance of the campaign. You also should make use of multiple channels of communication, including social media. In addition to traditional print, video, and online promotions, consider developing and using specially tailored apps, both for use by insiders during the campaign and for the general public as the campaign moves forward.

Finally, remember that while donors will be drawn in by emotion, before writing a check or signing a pledge card, they will want to be assured your plan has been carefully thought out.

People

Woody Hayes, a popular Ohio State University college football coach, is credited with saying you "win with people." Hayes recognized people make the biggest difference in success. People are the one resource that makes a true difference to a campaign success. They are the prime dynamic any campaign has, and this is the key principle behind fundraising success and differentiation. It is a well-known theory in fundraising circles that people give to people, to urgent and compelling causes, to campaigns when they have been invited to provide input and advice, and to campaigns when they have the opportunity to participate in the decision-making process. They do not give to causes that seem unimportant to them, that are poorly planned or managed, or that are ineffectively communicated.

The hospital will not be successful in a campaign without a high-quality team of people to implement, execute, and invest.

1. Enlist Internal Hospital Leadership Support

Philanthropy must be well-positioned internally and have the advocacy and support of key leaders within the hospital's senior management. Internal clarity amongst these parties about the vision for the campaign leads to effective external outreach. Within a hospital, there are four critical fundraising influencers:

Chief Executive Officer

The hospital chief executive officer (CEO) is regarded as the chief representative of a hospital's fundraising campaign due to the importance placed on this high-profile leader in the mind of donors. The CEO is respected by staff, board, donors, clients, vendors, and the larger community and must be willing to commit time to working on the campaign. Naturally, the CEO must set aside time to be involved in donor cultivation during a campaign; this is a key responsibility of the CEO. There will be myriad meetings, lunches, cocktail parties, and early-morning breakfasts at which the CEO will play a prominent role with groups large and small. The CEO is uniquely positioned to best communicate with major and top-level donors who will be looking for time with the CEO before making a major commitment. The CEO's time is a finite resource, so make calendaring and time management of the CEO a top priority.

Senior Management Team

The hospital senior management team should help pave the road to success by helping cultivate a culture of philanthropy. They are responsible for attaching importance and showing how they, as leaders, appreciate an environment where everyone in the hospital recognizes the value of the philanthropic dollar. They should explain the importance of philanthropy and how employees under their management can get involved. Equally importantly, all of these hospital leaders should personally contribute to the campaign.

Among all of the senior management leaders, the hospital chief financial officer (CFO) is probably the next most valuable internal ally to the CEO. A hospital CFO who truly understands the potential of philanthropy as part of the larger financial mix is very valuable, especially because the language of accounting and fundraising is somewhat different. Having a collaborative CFO who understands not only why investment in fundraising operations is important, but also what constitutes fundraising performance, is a tremendous asset.

Clinical Leaders

Physicians and nurses are instrumental to a hospital's campaign success. They often have the closest relationships with some of the potential biggest donors: grateful patients. Early on, fundraising staff should meet with physicians and educate them on the goals of the campaign, request contributions, and advise them on how they might encourage patients to contribute or at least meet with fundraising staff, who can get these patients more engaged with the hospital and begin cultivating them as donors.

Engagement of clinical leaders in hospital campaigns is consistent with the HIPAA Privacy rule that governs the appropriate use of protected patient information. Hospitals can appropriately do targeted fundraising based on the nature of the clinical services a patient received or the identity of his or her physician. In addition, employment of physicians by hospitals has sharply increased in the past few years, creating a pipeline of physician fundraising advocates. It behooves us to enlighten them as part of their onboarding about their role in assisting in the pursuit of philanthropic support for the hospital.

Fundraising Staff

A strong fundraising team is the foundation of any successful campaign effort and can't be overlooked as the very first and perhaps most valuable *people* element of launching a successful campaign. The staff should be viewed as partners with senior management and physician leaders in achieving fundraising goals. Proper staffing for a campaign is critical. No matter what the size of the hospital and the development staff, consideration must be given to the amount of time the campaign will take from current staff and the needs for adding staff. If building a team for a campaign, adopt a philosophy to hire very smart people who can come in and quickly gain the respect and trust of hospital executives, clinicians, and volunteer leaders.

2. Utilize Strong Leadership Volunteers

The importance of volunteers—particularly committed, high-capacity, enthusiastic volunteer leaders—simply cannot be overstated. Among the many decisions to be made in planning a campaign, selection of the best volunteer leadership is the single greatest factor for determining overall success. The most effective leaders will become involved because of their commitment to and interest in the hospital's campaign and not solely because of their wealth, connections, or willingness to lend their name. Their commitment should encompass several things:

- Belief in the mission,
- A sincere desire to serve others and the community, and
- A capacity to communicate those values to others and inspire them to become involved.

Among the leadership volunteers, there are three prominent influencers:

Governing Board

The hospital governing board alone is the activating force for any campaign, and their commitment is essential before undertaking a campaign. The board holds the power to approve or disapprove hospital programs and projects and any corresponding fundraising activity because they are the primary stewards of the hospital. And if the board approves the expenditure of funds for a hospital program or project, they must agree to the parallel responsibility of raising the funds and giving generously themselves. They must also participate in the solicitation of others. In all cases, 100% board giving to the campaign should be required before asking for public support. The presence of board members at key campaign events will be required to show their united support of this project. Preparing for a campaign often starts with the beefing up of a hospital board in advance of the campaign. Finally, the hospital board chair should be viewed as a strong, influential voice to support and advance the campaign and the entire philanthropic agenda.

Campaign Planning Committee

A dedicated and enthusiastic campaign planning committee is essential to a successful campaign. These high-level volunteers provide early credibility and undertake essential relationship-building to attract early campaign advocates and supporters both internally and in the community. They assist in steering the feasibility-study process; building belief in the importance, urgency, and value of the campaign; and providing early feedback on which programs, opportunities, and projects are the most compelling to potential donors.

Campaign Cabinet

Once the governing board has concurred with the feasibility study recommendation to proceed, the next step is to put together a well-connected, hardworking campaign cabinet to oversee the campaign. The planning committee may naturally evolve into a campaign cabinet, but beyond these members, the committee should include members of the board, appropriate clinical staff, and other philanthropists and volunteers from the community who care about the hospital, understand the importance of the campaign, and have the time and willingness to see it to successful conclusion.

Take the time to choose carefully the cabinet's chair(s) and its members. Set sights high when recruiting; volunteer leaders must have respect and influence. They also must be enthusiastic about the campaign and willing to open doors to major donors and other volunteers. Above all, be patient, thorough, and highly selective, and do not worry about inviting too many who meet your qualifications to join. Lastly, all campaign cabinet members should be willing to lead by example and make a leadership pledge or gift. A leadership gift is not always judged solely by dollar amount. The timing of the pledge or contribution can also be significant. Lead gifts from cabinet members provide needed leverage and will significantly affect the strategy and timing for engaging other key volunteers who will propel the campaign to achieve its goal.

3. Engage Effectively with Current and Future Donors

A fundamental step in campaigning is to identify whom you will ask to support your hospital campaign. The three most important populations are:

Current Donors

Board members and development officers must be willing to develop the relationships and connections that already exist. Successful campaigns are not feasible without a pool of donors who already know and support the organization and would be willing to give at higher levels. Examine donor records or institutional memory to develop a catalog of potential donors by reviewing giving levels from past donors, exploring the top 10% of current donors, and reviewing loyal donors who give annually. Expand your reach with donors in the middle of the giving pyramid. While a minority of lead donors may put a campaign on the map early on, engaging the many loyal mid-level donors will help you realize campaign success.

Pacesetter and Leadership Donors

Vilfredo Pareto was an Italian economist who, in the late 19th Century, created Pareto's Law, which states that 80% of the output is caused by 20% of the input. Simply put, 20% of the people will give 80% of the gifts. These are pacesetter and leadership donors. In hospital campaigns, you must focus on the 20% who can give 80% of the goal.

The well-known Sequence Solicitation principle states that gifts are solicited from the largest to the smallest gifts. This tenet is also applicable to campaigns. Always solicit from the top down and from

> The giving pyramid serves as a pictorial example to illustrate how donors are initially attracted by entry-level fundraising strategies at the base of the pyramid and cultivated over time to give larger gifts through successive engagement strategies. The pyramid reflects successive giving opportunities through which a donor is cultivated as the donor's commitment and capacity to assist an organization increases over time. The goal is to qualify current donors at each stage and encourage upward movement wherever appropriate.

the inside to the outside. Solicit your best and closest prospects first. Then move downward and outward to those who are your next best prospects. Eventually you will reach those who are farthest removed from your organization and who are prospects for the smallest gifts.

Prospects

It is well known that grateful patients and families are the best prospective donors for hospitals, primarily because they have the greatest understanding of a hospital's success in mission delivery. It is also well known that grateful patients and families will give to hospitals where they know people, where they have been deferentially treated, and where they are being kept informed of what's going on. To capture the opportunity grateful patients present, you should utilize an automated daily wealth screening of inpatients and outpatients, provide a high-quality service to high-capacity patients, and engage your physicians, nurses, and other hospital staff to thoughtfully connect with these potential donors. Indeed, *corporations, foundations,* and vendors are good prospective donors, and consideration must be given to them as well. However, stay especially focused on your efforts to engage grateful patients and their families. They will be the top prospects in your hospital campaign.

4. Embrace the Modern Ways People Connect to Each Other, Hospitals, and Fundraising Offices

To be successful with future campaigns, you need to embrace the ways people connect today. In recent years, there have been dramatic changes in how people use technology to connect and share experiences. Everything is increasingly integrated and "social": social media, social innovation, social networking, social entrepreneurs, and social philanthropy. Hospital donors will begin to see healthcare relationships in the same way they see their other relationships—as fully, and technologically, integrated into their daily lives.

Similarly, people will connect with our fundraising offices in very different ways. Technology must not be seen as a hindrance to human interaction. Instead, it is a tool to facilitate more individual, one-to-one, personalized experiences. The creation of gratifying gift experiences will be the essence of donor stewardship in healthcare campaigns of the future. Tomorrow's campaign donors will be interactive, get involved, and share information. We need to study how technology can be used to create high-touch, personalized donor experiences. Campaign offices need to be interconnected and utilize innovative technology to create unique, personal, high-touch experiences around campaigns. For example, with so many grateful patients (and potential donors) out there, it's hard for a hospital fundraising office to remember who has birthdays when, whose wedding anniversary is coming up, when a stewardship report is due, when the last acknowledgement letter was sent, and on and on. It is often difficult to stay on top of sending out a congratulatory card, stewardship report, or *Thank you* email. Technology will solve that problem. Software can automatically trigger reminders for a phone call or even send emails for you, keeping campaign donors happy and knowing that our thanking and staying in touch with them is our number-one priority. Embracing this new, technological reality will be a key to success in campaigns of the future.

Pervasiveness

Fundraising for hospitals is no longer separable from the care provided; the foundation for it must be integrated into every touch point, through every provider and employee.

1. Build a Ubiquitous Philanthropic Culture

Culture influences everything that goes on in a hospital. Best-practice hospitals achieve success in fundraising campaigns by creating a pervasive philanthropic culture. Although hard to define and difficult to put a finger on, culture is extremely powerful. It is the underground stream of values, beliefs, traditions, and rituals that have built up over time as people work together and resolve challenges, shaping how people think, feel, and act. This prevailing web of influence binds hospitals, volunteers, and the community together and makes it special. Hospital leaders—CEO, senior management team, physicians, nurses, fundraising staff, and volunteer leaders—must all commit to building a positive philanthropic culture. Without a pervasive and supportive culture of philanthropy, campaigns can weaken and stall.

2. Promote Philanthropy Everywhere the Hospital Brand Appears

These days, hospitals care for individuals across a much broader range of settings and circumstances. We must promote our campaigns and expand grateful patient prospecting strategies across the entire care continuum. We do this by partnering with care providers in all care locations; casting a wider net to understand the prospect opportunities in all settings, such as performing daily wealth screening on outpatient appointments; and appreciating our community's relationship with our entire brand of services and locations.

Passion

There can be little argument that passion is a valuable campaigning asset. It is what drives the campaign forward. To achieve success, you need to create a pervasive philanthropic culture. But pervasiveness alone is not enough; there must be passion in your entire hospital for the campaign.

1. Create Passion within Your Hospital

To organize a positive campaign, you need to truly impassion the entire organization about the need for philanthropic investment. You need to empower all hospital employees to get involved, showing them how their work impacts the hospital and the community. The entire hospital staff, not just the fundraisers, must be passionate in order for the community to be passionate and to deploy that passion through giving. Promote, recognize, and celebrate employee acts of passion for the campaign.

2. Match Donor Passion with Hospital Priorities

Finding donors' passions is the key to getting them to invest. Donors give when they have an emotional stake in, or philanthropic passion for, the mission of the hospital. Fundraisers have often been described as matchmakers because they strive to build relationships that will be long-lasting and mutually satisfying. Good fundraisers are donor-centered, supportive, and caring. They know that, as in human relationships, they simply cannot force a match; the connection must be natural. Really talented fundraisers bring donors together with hospital priorities during a campaign. They learn about a donor's passions and match them with campaign priorities.

Persistence

A good campaigner is persistent. Campaigning takes time, effort, and dedication to reach your goals. No matter how prepared you are, you will face roadblocks and adversity while on your campaign journey. You simply cannot give up, and there are no shortcuts. You must be in it for the long haul and remain singularly focused and committed to reaching the final destination.

1. Run a Marathon, Not a Sprint

Campaigns are like running a marathon, but too many people start out at a sprint. They get out of the gates quickly; experience some short-term success with a few leadership-level, low-hanging fruit gifts; and build some momentum. The problem comes when they face their first serious roadblock, such as when a gift they have worked hard on doesn't close for the amount projected. They get tripped up at the first real obstacle and then lose all the momentum they've achieved. They give up and quit at the first struggle, the first sign of volunteer transition or fatigue, the first sign of stalling. And they consequently leave their dreams unrealized. All of this can be avoided with proper mindset.

By treating the campaign like a marathon, you'll be prepared to overcome obstacles on your way to success. Even though you may get frustrated or fatigued, with the proper perspective, you will keep plugging away and moving in the right direction. Then, when you least expect it, instead of coming upon another obstacle, you instead receive an important gift that slingshots you forward. You must always keep pushing forward—especially when it is hardest.

In a campaign, there will be times when you feel like you are running straight uphill into a headwind. But you can be assured there will be times of celebration when the wind is at your back and it feels like you are running downhill. If you practice persistence and stay the course to finish strong, you will reach the great success your hospital strives to achieve.

2. Be Agile to Anticipate and Absorb Change

These days, a number of hospital strategic plans waver and remain ambiguous as reform-related imperatives delay judgments on priorities and long-term decision making. Hospital strategic priorities, and the capital projects associated with them, have become increasingly subject to unexpected and sometimes sweeping change. The volatile economic environment and evolving national healthcare agenda have accelerated variation. Campaign structures must attempt to be more agile to anticipate and absorb changes in funding priorities. The ability to foresee and manage change has clearly become a key competency for campaigns. Given these inevitable and frequent shifts in priorities, fundraising teams must establish more flexible campaign structures— without making worse the cycle of staff and volunteer burnout. Until the proverbial dust settles, campaign plans of the future will be much stronger if they incorporate change principles into the plan and continually revisit them.

Conclusion

Most hospitals think of campaign success in terms of the dollars raised, but a successful campaign goes far beyond the money. The real purpose of a campaign is to improve your hospital's overall health. You must judge success not only by the financial results of a specific campaign but also by the transformation of a hospital into one that can continue to enjoy robust fundraising both now and in the future. Never forget that, at the end of the day, it's about mission, message, and then money—from the donor perspective. Remember to celebrate small and big victories. Celebration can be a way to recognize and thank volunteers and donors, show off your accomplishment to the broader community, and brand your hospital with success.

Undoubtedly, today's healthcare environment calls for new, advanced, and adjusted fundraising approaches and campaign designs. But in changing times like these, consideration on timeless ingredients is even more valuable than it is in stable times. The five essential ingredients of the Campaign Mix are preparation, people, pervasiveness, passion, and persistence. When these five ingredients are mixed together and properly balanced, a hospital will achieve great success in a capital campaign.

Executive Summary

The Campaign Mix encompasses the 5 *P*'s of successful hospital capital campaigning and includes:

Preparation
- Align with the hospital's strategic plan
- Explore opportunities beyond bricks and mortar
- Establish the length and scope of the effort
- Conduct a feasibility study
- Create a captivating case for support

People
- Enlist internal hospital leadership support
- Utilize strong leadership volunteers
- Engage effectively with current and future donors
- Embrace the modern ways people connect to each other, hospitals, and fundraising offices

Pervasiveness
- Build a ubiquitous philanthropic culture
- Promote philanthropy everywhere the hospital brand appears

Passion
- Create passion within your hospital
- Match donor passion with hospital priorities

Persistence
- Run a marathon, not a sprint
- Be agile to anticipate and absorb change

Discussion Questions

A good way to understand the 5 *P*'s is through the questions that you need to ask to define your Campaign Mix. Here are some questions that will help you understand and define each of the five ingredients:

Preparation

Do you have a hospital strategic plan that has been prepared by senior staff in collaboration with the fundraising office and has been approved by the board?

People

Will the hospital CEO and senior management team give their full support to the fundraising during the period of the campaign?

Pervasiveness

Are you promoting your campaign and expanding grateful patient prospecting strategies across your entire care continuum?

Passion

Are you impassioning and empowering all hospital employees to get involved in your campaign and showing them how their work impacts the hospital mission and community?

Persistence

Are you incorporating change principles and flexibility into your campaign plan?

While the questions I have listed above are important, they are just a subset of the detailed probing that may be required to optimize your Campaign Mix.

Author Bio

Bill Mountcastle is the founder and president of Health Philanthropy Services Group, LLC. He has more than two decades of experience in fundraising, rising to senior leadership positions at leading multi-specialty academic medical centers and research universities with sophisticated and successful development programs. Prior to his founding Health Philanthropy Services Group, Mountcastle served in capital campaign leadership positions at Cleveland Clinic, University Hospitals, and The Ohio State University. He has directed fundraising programs to support capital campaign projects, medical education, patient care, and research activities for main campus hospitals, regional operations, and national and international programs.

End of One Size Fits All!
The Past and the Promise of
Cross-Cultural Philanthropy
Lilya Wagner, CFRE

Bᴀᴄᴋ ᴀᴛ ᴛʜᴇ ᴛᴜʀɴ ᴏꜰ ᴛʜᴇ ᴄᴇɴᴛᴜʀʏ, and even before, eminent lead-ers in the nonprofit and philanthropic sector were asking, "Why does everyone suddenly care about diverse donor groups? Why is everyone suddenly interested in diversity in philanthropy and fundraising? Why is identity-based philanthropy getting so much attention?" Perhaps the answers lie in some of the following statements.

- The world has grown increasingly conscious of cultural diversity as population shifts have occurred, repres-sive governments have failed and in some cases disap-peared, and minorities have found a voice through civil society, nonprofit organizations, or nongovernmental organizations.[83]
- These very organizations have become increasingly aware that they will raise more money, have more community

---

83 A non-governmental organization (NGO) is a legally constituted organization created by natural or legal person that operates independently from any form of government. The term originated from the United Nations (UN), and is normally used to refer to organiza-tions that are not a part of the government and are not conventional for-profit business.

support, and be able to more effectively carry out their
missions—if they take cultural diversity and philanthropy
into account.

- The nonprofit sector everywhere, but especially in the
Western Hemisphere, has grown increasingly conscious
that one size no longer fits all—that services to diverse
population groups must be adapted culturally; and,
therefore, fundraising must also take place with cultural
consciousness in mind.

Until the late '80s or early '90s, North America was paying little
attention to cultural differences when it came to nonprofit sustainability through philanthropic means, and neither was much of the rest of
the world, where formal fundraising practice was just getting a toehold.
And yet, as an eminent figure in the foundation world, Emmett Carson
wrote in 2000, "It is important to state at the outset that donors of
color are not new donors. Quite the contrary; many racial and ethnic
groups have charitable giving traditions that predate the founding of
North America..."[84] He goes on to state that the old rules of donor
engagement hamper efforts to solicit diverse donor groups and that
new rules can help nonprofits raise funds and other support from these
prospective donors much more effectively.

So while conversations about diversity in philanthropy and fundraising were burgeoning, and research was gaining prominence and
informing the nonprofit world, Royster Hedgepeth wrote in 2002,
"Philanthropy and fundraisers are at the crossroads. Where do these
roads lead? Who is on the road with us? What tools do we need to
succeed? How will we know we have arrived?"[85]

The time has been right to ask questions about diversity in the nonprofit sector, especially when it comes to programs, services, and the funds

---

84 Emmett Carson. "The New Rules for Engaging Donors of Color: Giving in the Twenty-
First Century," New Directions for Philanthropic Fundraising (Bloomington, IN: John
Wiley & Sons, 2000): 69.

85 Royster C. Hedgepeth, "Spanning Boundaries and Building Bridges," New Directions
for Philanthropic Fundraising (Bloomington, IN: John Wiley & Sons, 2002): 117.

needed to develop, improve, and sustain these. Fortunately, for most in the sector, the discovery moment is past—the moment when we realize there really are differences in philanthropic preferences—and we can move forward with confidence that we have some answers, that we have a significant knowledge base in terms of research and practice, and that giving by diverse population groups—whether we call them minorities, people of color, identity-based, immigrants, or by their official ethnic title (*e.g.*, Mexicans or Ukranians)—is increasing as we truly realize that one size doesn't fit all when it comes to philanthropy and fundraising. Hedgepeth further wrote, "We know that there are differences between and among Caucasian, African-American, Asian, Hispanic, and Native American cultures regarding philanthropy and volunteerism. In our increasingly egalitarian society, the professional fundraiser needs to be able to move with confidence between and among these groups."[86]

Much progress has been made in awareness, in research-based practice that takes into account diversity, in cultural bases and biases, and in respect for differences in philanthropy, which guide differences in fundraising methods. Still, a report by the W. K. Kellogg Foundation noted as recently as 2012 that "Charitable giving in the US quickly is becoming more ethnically, culturally, and socioeconomically diverse, yet conventional philanthropy has not fully recognized, embraced, and partnered with communities of color and needs to understand and support their philanthropy if it wants to drive social change..."[87]

We now acknowledge that local roots that give modern philanthropy its impetus exist alongside Western ideas on how to motivate philanthropy that is based on ancient roots. As a 2009 article in *Advancing Philanthropy*, the journal of the Association of Fundraising Professionals stated, "Philanthropy among people of color is not new. People of color share a long, rich history of giving that has largely gone unnoticed because it does not fit the traditional image of philanthropy."[88] Building civil society

---

86 Hedgepeth, 109.

87 "Giving grows among communities of color," Philanthropy Journal, January 17, 2012, accessed January 29, 2013, http://www.philanthropyjournal.org/news/top-stories/ giving-grows-among-communities-color.

88 K. Lester, "A New Script," Advancing Philanthropy (March/April 2009): 11-13.

globally without reference to various traditions of philanthropy, whether in the country of origin or on a transnational basis, is incomplete and imbalanced. The author, Darryl Lester, suggests we need to change the philanthropy script "to broaden how philanthropists look, sound, and give."[89]

To not acknowledge, work with, and tap into diversity in North America and globally is to ignore much potential income for nonprofit healthcare organizations. This includes ethnic groups in North America who have brought cultural differences and traditions from many countries which shape their generosity and volunteerism, and this is true as population movements occur worldwide. To recognize that in the 21st century the philanthropy of women, communities of color, and youth are likely to have substantial influence on traditional philanthropic practices and institutions is to maximize the inclusivity inherent in giving and receiving funds for nonprofits. Fundraisers, therefore, find that in order to be successful, they must tailor their appeals to the prospective donors' customs and sensibilities.

What Hinders Progress in Cross-Cultural Philanthropy?

In an article by Sondra Thiederman written for *Training and Development*, she comments on "The Bias Burden." While the article is aimed at trainers and managers, her analysis and explanation readily applies to the healthcare fund development world: "It's sometimes our own biases, not those directed against us, that slow our professional progress."[90] Forms of bias can be many, as enumerated by the National Conference for Community and Justice:

- Exclusion and invisibility—these diminish the value given to particular groups and silence the legitimacy of their voices.
- Stereotyping—this portrays members of specific groups as having both negative and positive characteristics in common.

89 Lester, 11-13.
90 Sondra Thiederman, "The Bias Burden," T+D Magazine (August 2004): 50.

- Imbalance and selectivity—presenting only one interpretation of an issue, situation, or group.
- Unreality—ignoring particular facts about groups or individuals because of prevailing beliefs, perceptions, or ideologies.
- Fragmentation and isolation—tendency to separate or isolate experiences of minority groups from those of the majority population.
- Linguistic bias—ethnic and racial slurs that aren't accurate but reinforce prevailing assumptions.[91]

Touré, a columnist for *TIME Magazine*, wrote that "bias is the complex neural interplay between emotions and beliefs."[92] He added that most people have some sort of prejudice or bias, which leads to discriminatory actions. While his examples deal with societal issues such as crime, the same concept can be applied to philanthropy and fundraising.

Perceptions about who can give, who will give, and what will be the focus of their support permeate nonprofit personnel attitudes ranging from leadership to fundraisers. These perceptions may be part of a natural human condition, but they are counterproductive in every way. Respect and acceptance of differences can enrich both individual and collective experience and also, when it comes to nonprofits and the philanthropy that supports them, result in greater viability and sustainability of the organizations that make up our civil societies.

Therefore fund development personnel who work for nonprofit healthcare organizations should avail themselves of information that leads to a greater awareness of philanthropic traditions that dictate practice, resulting in greater inclusivity in carrying out the nonprofit mission.

---

91 Richard Koonce, "Redefining Diversity," T+D Magazine (August 2004): 50.
92 Touré, "Inside the Racist Mind," TIME Magazine, April 19, 2012, 20.

Defining Philanthropy in a Cross-Cultural Context

According to the founding director of the Center on Philanthropy at Indiana University, Robert L. Payton, philanthropy can be defined as "voluntary action for the public good."[93] This may be a comfortable definition for Americans, but different interpretations of the term *philanthropy* exist among populations, cultures, and countries. The philanthropic preferences and actions of various populations, both in the US and globally, result in various definitions and interpretations, causing both a richness that translates into a practice of generosity and also a confusion of terms and their meanings. In the UK, for examples, the terms *charity* and *philanthropy* are often interchangeable, while for many minorities *philanthropy* doesn't apply to them but only to rich, white folks. Even in the United States, confusion about the word *philanthropy* is prevalent and assumed to be the domain of the well-known wealthy like Microsoft founder Bill Gates.

However, when considering diverse population groups, the term *philanthropy* may need to be explained and defined in local cultural contexts. It's even possible that euphemisms must be adopted, or the term must be adapted to local or regional use. Therefore, the healthcare fund development leader and practitioner should be conscious of language use as a whole and defining the concept of giving in particular. This, in turn, leads to considerations of diversity—diversity that is geographic, regional, cultural, experiential, and philanthropic.

For the purposes of this chapter, philanthropy is meant as the sharing of goods and services with no expectation of financial remuneration, particularly outside of the nuclear family.

---

93 "Philanthropy: Voluntary Action for the Public Good," accessed January 23, 2013, http://www.paytonpapers.org/book/index.shtm.

How Diversity Knowledge and Practice Informs Philanthropy

Companies are increasingly embracing diversity as a business expediency and a corporate value. They realize it isn't just the right thing to do. There's a strong, practical reason for embracing and practicing diversity because various and diverse population groups have increasing buying power. As stated in a publication of the Society for Human Resource Management, "Companies are experiencing an increased demand to adjust their fundamental practices to accommodate the cultural styles, norms, and preferences of the regions of the world where they operate. It has become an acceptable, even preferred in some cases, business practice to leverage the unique cultures and values that organizations bring from their national affiliation."[94]

A corollary to the corporate mentality regarding diversity is a nonprofit's acknowledgement that diversity in seeking funding support, both from the perspectives of the donor as well as the organization, is not just the right thing to do but is profitable for the cause. To paraphrase the above quotation about corporations and the need to embrace diversity, nonprofits are also experiencing an increased demand to adjust their fundamental practices to accommodate the cultural styles, norms, and preferences of the regions of the world where they operate. The nonprofit synergies that can be brought to bear through global organizational alignment often produce superior humanitarian results in comparison to a non-global approach. Yet not all organizations have embraced diversity from this perspective, even though the for-profit sector has seen the wisdom in its application of theory.

Diversity goes much beyond acknowledging and including ethnic groups, or diverse populations, or minorities—depending on how one wishes to define differences. And perhaps attitudes that view diversity quite narrowly could be excused because it does take some effort to

---

94 Vanessa J. Weaver and Shawn Coker, "Globalization and Diversity," Mosaics, SHRM Focuses on Workplace Diversity (2000): 1.

become sensitive to differing communication styles, different concepts of time, and different loyalties to nonprofit causes.

If we are to take diversity seriously as a value that shapes our philanthropic practice, we must define diversity itself. Diversity is not synonymous with differences but encompasses differences and similarities. Diversity refers to different cultural identities, ideas, and work functions, and it isn't just about people. An expert in fundraising and ethics, Marilyn Fischer, stated that "understanding and valuing diversity involves both equity and ethics." She pointed out the many ways to think about the basic equality of all people, including treating people in a manner that respects their intrinsic worth and dignity. Furthermore, the ethics of prejudice include perceptual inequities that occur when people misunderstand and therefore misjudge others.[95]

When defining how various businesses approach diversity, the international consulting firm Deloitte's national managing director of human resources stated that "we go beyond the usual things to talk about, things like value system, language, geographic experience and location, working style, thinking style, educational background, involvement in the military, socioeconomic class, religion, all the things that make up the dynamics of who we are."[96] The proactive healthcare development professional would do well to consider this approach to diversity in enabling philanthropy from diverse population groups; it certainly is similar to excellent prospect-research practices with the cultural layer as a prominent feature.

Fortunately, many nonprofit organizations are embracing diversity as a mission and organizational value. They are seeking to tap into the economic growth and power of Hispanics, African-Americans, Asian-Americans, and other diverse population groups. Reis and Clohesy, in writing about the "new donor" of the 21st century, stated, "As these populations grow in numbers, they will continue to grow in influence and resources. In the 21st century the philanthropy of women,

---

95 Marilyn Fischer, "Respecting the Individual, Valuing Diversity," Critical Issues in Fund Raising, ed. Dwight F. Burlingame, (New York: John Wiley & Sons, Inc., 1997): 65-71.
96 Molly Rose Teuke, "Rethinking Diversity," Continental, March 2003, 44.

communities of color, and youth are likely to have a substantial influence on traditional philanthropic institutions. Already these populations have created new philanthropic institutions and networks that more closely resemble their social/ethnic cultures and attempt to solve issues they consider to be of most importance."[97]

One of the challenges in achieving diversity in philanthropy is the use of language. Even the commonly used phrase "fundraising in diverse communities," often found in titles of books and articles, can be disputed. Perhaps it would be more correct to say, "fundraising across, within, among, for, or with diverse communities." The descriptive term that has become most acceptable is identity-based philanthropy.

A group of fundraisers identified the special meanings the word *diversity* had for them, and these can serve as our transition point to considering culture and philanthropy.

"Diversity is about maximizing resources all across the entire organization."

"Diversity should weave through everything we talk about; it's not a separate topic."

"Diversity is reaching out to forgotten populations."

"Diversity is about how society is changing. It is spiritual growth for a whole society."

"Take diversity and translate it into fundraising—that's what we're really talking about when we reach beyond our own backyards to develop new resources."[98]

---

97 Thomas K. Reis and Stephanie J. Clohesy, "Unleashing New Resources and Entrepreneurship for the Common Good: A Philanthropic Renaissance," Foundations in Europe, (Bertelsmann Foundation, June 2000): 12.

98 "Multicultural Organizational Development," Advancing Philanthropy (January/February 2012): 57.

Cultural Foundations for Fundraising

Primary to any discussion of diverse populations, a consideration of what culture means is valuable for providing a foundation or framework. According to Wilson, "Culture strongly influences how one behaves and how one understands the behavior of others, and cultures vary in the behaviors they find proper and acceptable."[99] There is the external culture, which is exhibited in outward behaviors and traditions that are readily discernible, such as a performance of a mariachi band, and internal culture, which is less evident, such as the way people think about situations and conceptualize information. Culture is a complex phenomenon. To summarize, it might be best to say that culture is to a group what personality is to an individual.

In applying these qualities to the relationship between culture and philanthropy, the authors of *Philanthropy in Communities of Color* explained culture in this way: "All cultures construct reality differently; within each unique cultural community, beliefs and behavior have meanings that are often not shared or understood by the outside world. Some cultural meanings are manifest and easily recognized; others are latent and subtle, requiring systematic observation in order to produce accurate analysis."[100]

Consequently, a consideration of cultural elements is vital prior to any fundraising activity. The authors of *Philanthropy in Communities of Color* also stated that "the cultural dimensions of gift-giving, financial assistance, sharing, and the distribution of income and wealth all have a variety of meanings from culture to culture... The uses of wealth, prestige, and power are also important to the cross-cultural analysis of charitable behavior."[101]

---

99 Meena. S. Wilson, Michael. H. Hoppe, and Leonard. R. Sayles, *Managing Across Cultures: A Learning Framework* (Greensboro, NC: Center for Creative Leadership, 1996), 1.

100 Bradford S. Smith, Sylvia Shue, Jennifer. L. Vest & Joseph Villarreal. *Philanthropy in Communities of Color*. (Bloomington, IN: Indiana University Press, 1999): 3.

101 ibid

In *Racial, Ethnic and Tribal Philanthropy: A Scan of the Landscape,*[102] the authors suggest that cultural competence is fundamental to understanding and supporting philanthropic engagement. Cultural competence suggests an awareness of one's own culture and awareness and acceptance of others' cultures. In an effort to improve cultural competence, a Cultural Competence Learning Initiative was launched by San Francisco-based CompassPoint Nonprofit Services. Elements identified as building blocks for developing cultural competency in a nonprofit included clarifying assumptions about cultural differences, management's commitment to multi-culturalism, shifting cultural norms and candid conversations on topics sometimes shunned, codifying and articulating assumptions, and taking responsibility for change, both internal and external.[103]

Unfortunately, many fundraisers approach a relationship and solicitation from their own perspective, therefore leaving themselves unprepared for cultural differences that can easily be misinterpreted and misconstrued. Perspectives of other cultures may be inaccurate, yet these must be corrected. As described in a *Harvard Business Review* article which addressed "Three Skills every 21st Century Manager Needs," such action calls for "code switching between cultures." The author defined this as the ability to modify behavior, to accommodate various cultural norms, and to have a capacity to manage the psychological challenges that arise when cultural knowledge is translated into action.[104]

Among the cultural challenges presented to the nonprofit executive and fundraiser is terminology. Should correct designation for diverse populations other than Anglos be *people of color, minorities,* or *ethnic groups*? And is the correct terminology *African-American* or *black*? *Hispanic* or *Latino*? *Asian-American,* and/or *Pacific Islander*? Just possibly, labels get in the way more than they help when we identify and qualify donors.

102 K. R. Lindsey, Racial, Ethnic, and Tribal Philanthropy: A Scan of the Landscape (Washington, D.C.: Forum of Regional Associations of Grantmakers, 2006).

103 "Multicultural Organizational Development," 57.

104 Andrew L. Molinsky, "Three Skills every 21st Century Manager Needs," Harvard Business Review (January/February 2012): 140.

Naturally, people of diverse populations would prefer to be identified by their actual country of origin, or their source of national orientation. Mexicans or Mexican-Americans, for example, would rather be distinctive than lumped into an overall designation. Chinese may have few similarities with Pacific Islanders, yet they usually come under the same appellation. The term *people of diverse populations* appears to be becoming the term of preference. Although *people of color* has commonly been used, more objections have been noted in recent years to this designation.

Overview of Cross-Cultural Giving

Having addressed diversity and culture, we then come to the question of how people give and why people behave in altruistic ways. Giving by diverse population groups, or identity-based philanthropy, is nothing new. Our understanding, however, of how and why such donors give is growing. In 2006, an article in *Philanthropy Journal* stated, "Diverse donors giving back: Racial ethnic and tribal philanthropy growing rapidly."[105] The article concluded that the face of the US is changing and with it, the face of philanthropy. The changing face, of course, brought with it the cultural influences and traditions from countries of origin, whether first generation or further back, and therefore dictated how philanthropy also has changed. Along with this positive fact, however, comes a challenge that diverse donors pose. "'Donors in the US have become more diverse, and charities need to work harder to understand and engage them,' experts say."[106]

However, some myths persist, and among these is that minorities, or people of color, don't give. This has been a tenet of US fundraising that, fortunately, is rapidly being dispelled. We must acknowledge, of course, that sometimes giving occurs in ways that the nonprofit world or the IRS doesn't recognize, and much giving is informal and doesn't adhere to the model developed by Caucasian males, who were instrumental in

---

105 Ellen Barclay and Barry Gaberman, "Diverse Donors Giving Back," Philanthropy Journal, accessed December 18, 2006. http://www.philanthropyjournal.org/archive/124184.

106 Todd Cohen, "Diverse donors pose challenges," Philanthropy Journal, accessed October 30, 2007, http://www.philanthropyjournal.org/resources/special-reports/fundraising/diverse-donors-pose-challenges.

establishing philanthropy on American soil and founded many influential organizations as America was settled and developed. In "The Roots of Minority Giving," M. Ann Abbe points out that these models don't reflect the true amount of philanthropy in other cultures because minorities do not give for the same reasons or in the same manner.[107] While education, wealth, community involvement, and other characteristics and activities are increasing among minorities, the question no longer is whether or not fundraisers should engage minorities but *how*.

For most minority communities, philanthropy is viewed in a broad sense that includes time, talent, and money, and donations are made without fanfare or concern about records or reporting. Often gifts are unplanned and unrecognized, and they revolve around family, church, and education. While generalizations should be approached with caution because these do not capture everyone in a defined population group, generalizations can serve as a starting point for noting what to notice—what might be unique characteristics in certain categories of generosity behaviors that a fundraiser should observe and therefore adjust the funding request appropriately. Abbe points these out:

- Direct, informal support to children, the elderly, or community members is more common than support of institutions.
- Level of immediate need is a major consideration in giving. Immediate needs take precedence over long-term planning.
- Planned giving is seldom a priority.
- There is some distrust of traditional nonprofit institutions related to a perception that these have not met minority needs.
- There is some distrust of traditional forms of giving.
- Individual cultures within minority groups do not always agree on philanthropic priorities and interests because of their varying histories and experiences.[108]

---

107 Maura King Scully, "Untangling," CASE Currents (July/August 2000): 35-41.
108 M. Ann Abbe, "Untangling," CASE Currents (July/August 2000): 35-41.

Adding to these the effect of recentness of immigration versus long-term stay in the US or other countries, as well as diaspora, philanthropy causes astute nonprofit leaders and personnel, including fundraisers, to perhaps feel a weight of "too much to know." But experience now indicates that these cultural differences in practicing philanthropy must be considered in successful fundraising programs.

As a report in *Philanthropy Journal* stated, "Giving grows among communities of color," cultural differences in philanthropy can hardly be ignored.[109] Not heeding the ways in which diverse communities give is neglecting significant groups or individual donors who can add to the sustainability of a nonprofit.

Business as Unusual— Culture and Diversity in Philanthropy

"Nonprofit groups seeking to tap the growing economic power of Blacks, Hispanics, and Asian-Americans should tailor their fundraising appeals to the prospective donors' customs and sensibilities…"[110] "Making assumptions about donors' backgrounds is widespread, and charities should work harder to overcome preconceived notions of ethnicity when dealing with minority donors…"[111] "Development officers must retool and refine their outreach efforts."[112]

Statements like these are a wakeup call to nonprofits in the US as well as elsewhere. As a popular warning sign says, "Ignore at your own peril." So a cautionary approach could be advisable for nonprofit personnel who fail to embrace the cultural richness of their potential constituents and donors.

---

109 "Giving Grows Among Communities of Color," January 17, 2012, accessed January 29, 2013, http://www.philanthropyjournal.org/news/top-stories/giving-grows-among-communities-color.

110 Emmett Carson, as quoted by Michael Anft, "Raising Money With Sense and Sensibility," Philanthropy Journal, October 18, 2001, accessed January 29, 2013, http://philanthropy.com/article/Raising-Money-With-Sense-an/52257/.

111 Janice G. Pettey as quoted by Michael Anft, "Raising Money With Sense and Sensibility," Philanthropy Journal, October 18, 2001, accessed January 29, 2013, http://philanthropy.com/article/Raising-Money-With-Sense-an/52257/.

112 Michele Collison, "Beyond Borders," CASE Currents (January 2004): 16-22.

Consider a few suggestions on a philanthropic script:

Step 1: Broaden the definition of philanthropy to be more inclusive of the traditions of giving among diverse populations.

Step 2: Revive the concept of community philanthropy and the spirit of collective giving that is central to changing the "philanthropic script."[113]

A review of the literature in fundraising among diverse populations indicates that traditional fundraising principles have to be adapted to changing donor populations. The fundraising professional needs to consider variations on donor approaches, including one-on-one solicitation, direct mail, use of the Internet, and telephone solicitation. Prospect research strategies must be redefined to capture information that is relevant and suitable to diverse donor identification and cultivation. Volunteers representing various ethnic groups will need to be recruited and trained.

Perhaps prior to an organization's modifying or enhancing its fundraising strategies and practices, however, is for that organization to commit to diversity, both internally and among constituents and donors; to modify its organizational mission to reflect this commitment; and to provide any necessary training or programs that create awareness of diversity issues. To accomplish this, an organization must have top-level leadership support as well as diversity in its ranks. A needs statement should be crafted, which identifies the organization's status regarding diversity, its willingness to embrace diversity, and how diversity issues fit into the organization framework. Focus groups can provide excellent feedback and advice. From there, best practices can be developed through study and research, and a transformational program can be established.

Nonprofit healthcare organizations have a stellar opportunity to increase giving from diverse groups now and in the coming years. This fact provides organizations with numerous opportunities to

---

113 Lester, "A New Script," 11-13.

understand and interact with rich differences in languages, values, and cultural practices. It is a movement away from homogenizing everyone to accepting and embracing cultural richness in our lives.

Executive Summary

- Culture influences how generosity is practiced.
- In the United States, as in much of the rest of the world, generosity has existed throughout history yet has seen a resurgence in formalized philanthropy in recent decades for various political as well as migratory reasons.
- Understanding identity-based philanthropy, what motivates giving, and how fundraisers should relate to differences in practices and attitudes about generosity is vital for successful nonprofits, both in relating to their constituents as well as their potential and current donors.

Discussion

1. What aspects of culture most influence philanthropic action, regardless of the country and/or society under consideration?

2. How does time spent living in a specific country affect retention of cultural differences in generosity versus assimilation into and absorption of practices and attitudes of the country of residence?

3. What are the realities today of how nonprofits relate to differences as exhibited by identity-based constituents and donors? How does YOUR organization handle these differences when it comes to fundraising?

4. What are the key points that a fundraising professional should know and remember when approaching donors who are not mainstream?

5. What are the best, most recommended ways to acquire information about identity-based donors, particularly when they are different from one's own perspectives and experiences?

Author Bio

Dr. Lilya Wagner is director of Philanthropic Service for Institutions and is on the faculty of the Indiana University Lilly Family School of Philanthropy. During 14 years of association with the Center on Philanthropy at Indiana University, she served as associate director of The Fund Raising School and director of the Women's Philanthropy Institute. She is a frequent author; her published writings include articles and book chapters on philanthropy, fundraising, and the nonprofit sector.